The Electromyographer's Handbook

The Electromyographer's Handbook

Second Edition

Rajesh K. Sethi, M.D., M.R.C.P.(U.K.)
*Formerly Clinical Research Fellow in
Neurophysiology, Harvard Medical School and
Brigham and Women's Hospital, Boston; Director,
Electromyography Laboratory, Marquette General
Hospital, Marquette*

Lowery Lee Thompson, M.D.
*Clinical Associate Professor of Family Medicine and
Comprehensive Care, Louisiana State University
School of Medicine in Shreveport; Neurology
Associates, Monroe*

Little, Brown and Company
Boston/Toronto

To my son, Neeruj

Library of Congress Catalog Card No. 88-83898

ISBN 0-316-84187-0

Printed in the United States of America

HAL

Contents

Preface   *vii*
Acknowledgments   *ix*

1 *Introduction to Nerve Conduction Studies*   *1*
2 *Brachial Plexus: Motor Studies*   *22*
3 *Ulnar Nerve: Motor and Sensory Studies*   *31*
4 *Median Nerve: Motor and Sensory Studies*   *41*
5 *Radial Nerve: Motor and Sensory Studies*   *49*
6 *Musculocutaneous Nerve: Sensory Studies*   *56*
7 *Sciatic Nerve, Lumbosacral Roots, and Plexus: Motor Studies*   *59*
8 *Peroneal Nerve: Motor Studies*   *67*
9 *Superficial Peroneal Nerve: Sensory Studies*   *72*
10 *Tibial Nerve: Motor and Sensory Studies*   *75*
11 *Sural Nerve: Sensory Studies*   *80*
12 *Femoral Nerve: Motor Studies*   *83*
13 *Saphenous Nerve: Sensory Studies*   *89*
14 *Facial Nerve: Direct Stimulation and Blink Reflex*   *92*
15 *The F-Wave*   *101*
16 *The H-Reflex*   *107*
17 *Repetitive Stimulation*   *114*
18 *The EMG Examination*   *123*
19 *Single Fiber Electromyography*   *152*
20 *Electrodiagnosis of Specific Neuromuscular Disorders*   *159*

Appendixes
I *Machine Settings for EMG and Nerve Conduction Studies*   *179*
II *Normal Values: Adults*   *180*
III *Normal Values: Children*   *182*
IV *Duration of Selected CMAPs*   *185*

V   *The Innervation of Commonly Studied Muscles by Named Nerves and Spinal Segments*   *186*

VI   *Myotomes of the Upper and Lower Extremities*   *187*

VII   *Motor Points of Commonly Studied Muscles*   *188*

Index   195

Preface

The second edition has undergone substantial revision of existing chapters and the addition of new ones to reflect the changes in the field of electrodiagnosis. The terminology conforms to the latest AAEE glossary of terms. The basic format with concise and practical text and numerous photographic illustrations and tables is unchanged. We hope the book will retain its appeal to beginners and practicing electromyographers alike.

The introductory chapter gives an overview of nerve conduction techniques. Great emphasis has been placed on technical details and the potential sources for errors.

The chapters on individual nerve conduction studies contain practical anatomic details and the electrodiagnostic set-up, accompanied by numerous photographic illustrations. An extensively revised data base of published normal values for individual nerves is tabulated and referenced. Graphs relating height to latency are provided for H-reflex and F-wave studies. The chapter on repetitive stimulation has been expanded to incorporate more details on the technique and correct interpretation of the results.

New techniques described include cervical and lumbosacral root stimulations, blink reflex, sympathetic skin response, ulnar dorsal cutaneous nerve study, plantar nerve study, tremor recordings, sphincter muscle studies, and single fiber EMG.

The final chapter contains concise and practical electrodiagnostic guidelines for the evaluation of specific neuromuscular disorders, and the electrophysiologic criteria used for their diagnosis.

The Appendixes are designed to serve as ready references for machine settings, normal values for adults and children, and for anatomic details most useful to the practicing electromyographer.

R. K. S.
L. L. T.

Acknowledgments

I would like to thank Dr. C. Krarup, Assistant Professor, Harvard Medical School and Director of the EMG laboratory at Brigham and Women's Hospital, Boston, who initiated me into this project and offered valuable suggestions throughout the preparation of this manuscript. I would like to personally acknowledge my gratitude to Dr. F. Bucthal, Dr. E. Stalberg, Dr. J. Kimura, Dr. D. Sanders, Dr. B. T. Shahani, Dr. R. I. Braddom, Dr. I. C. MacLean, Dr. W. Litchy, Dr. S. Oh, and Dr. C. Jablecki for permission to use their illustrations.

The assistance of Katherine Arnoldi and Laurie Anello, of Little, Brown and Company, is greatly appreciated; Alta Yancy, our technician, assisted with several studies; Peg Leahy coordinated the illustrations. Steve Shaw was responsible for the new drawings and Michael Adamian for the new photographic work. Last but not least I would like to acknowledge my enormous gratitude to my wife Malti, who helped to type the manuscript and was supportive throughout.

R. K. S.

The Electromyographer's Handbook

Introduction to Nerve Conduction Studies 1

Nerve conduction studies are commonly performed in the evaluation of suspected neuromuscular disease and provide an objective measure of pathophysiologic changes. With attention to technical detail, which is critical in arriving at reliable findings, results obtained in different laboratories are relatively consistent.

A brief description of the equipment and a general approach to the performance of nerve conduction studies are presented in this chapter; specific studies are detailed in the chapters that follow.

Apparatus

Figure 1-1 outlines the basic components of the apparatus used for nerve conduction studies, namely the electrodes, stimulator, amplifier, filters, display screen, and recording mechanism.

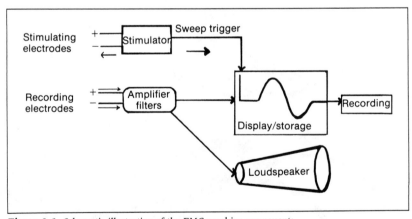

Figure 1-1. *Schematic illustration of the EMG machine components.*

Electrodes

A variety of surface electrodes are available, some of which are shown in Figure 1-2. The metal disc and ring electrodes can be used interchangeably for stimulating and recording. The impedance of the skin-electrode interface is reduced by cleaning the skin with acetone or alcohol and applying gel to the electrode. The electrodes are then firmly fixed to the skin with adhesive tape or a Velcro strap.

The *cathode* (color-coded black in all the illustrations) should always be closer to the active recording electrode (Fig. 1-3) except during

F-wave and H-reflex studies when the cathode points toward the spinal cord.

The *anode* (color-coded white in all the illustrations) is farther away from the active recording electrode (Fig. 1-3).

The *active recording electrode* (G_1, black for illustration purposes) is placed over the motor point of a muscle during motor nerve conduction studies (Fig. 1-3C) and over the nerve during sensory studies (Fig. 1-3A,B).

The *reference electrode* (G_2, white for illustration purposes) is placed distal to G_1 on the tendon during motor nerve conduction studies (Fig. 1-3C) and over the nerve during sensory studies (Fig. 1-3A,B).

The *ground electrode* (G_0) is usually placed between the stimulating and recording electrodes, close to G_1.

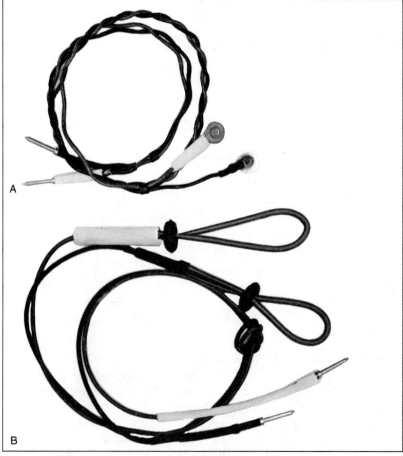

Figure 1-2. *Types of surface electrodes. The anode and G_2 electrodes are marked with white tape for clarity in the photographs. A. Small disc electrodes. B. Ring electrodes. C. Large disc electrode. D. Bipolar bar electrode. E. Bipolar stimulation electrode.*

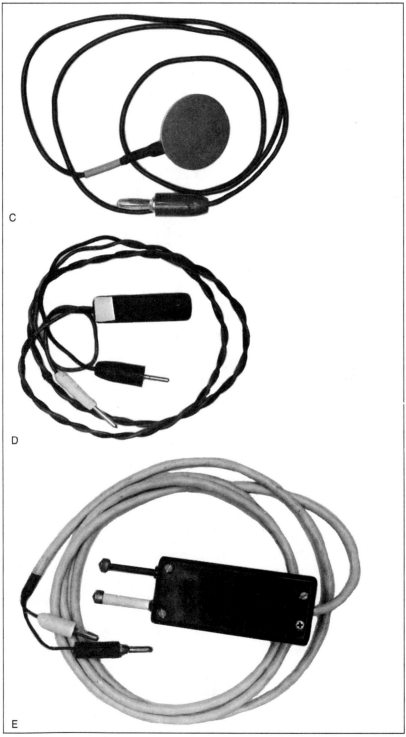

Figure 1-2. (Continued)

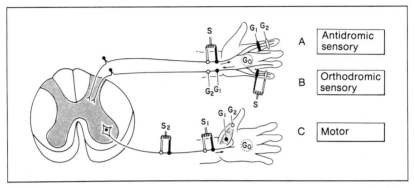

Figure 1-3. *Diagrammatic illustration of electrode placement for nerve conduction studies. Antidromic sensory study (A); orthodromic sensory study (B); and motor nerve conduction study (C). (G_1 = active recording electrode; G_2 = reference recording electrode; G_0 = ground electrode; S = stimulating electrode; S_1 = distal stimulation site; S_2 = proximal stimulation site. Cathode is black; anode is white.)*

Needle electrodes may be used for stimulating deep nerves such as the sciatic nerve. If a monopolar needle is used for stimulation then a surface disc electrode on the nearby skin is used as the anode (see Fig. 7-4).

Needle electrodes (see Fig. 18-1) are also used for recording from muscles that are deep or cannot be isolated (see Figs. 2-2 to 2-6).

Near nerve recordings (see Fig. 20-1) of nerve action potentials [1] are done with special stainless steel needle electrodes. The details of this technique are beyond the scope of this book, but the advantages are (1) a more precise onset of the potential, (2) the ability to record from more proximal sites where the nerves are less accessible to surface recording, (3) the ability to record very small potentials (<0.1 μV), and (4) a more accurate configuration of the potential and a better appreciation of dispersion (see Fig. 20-1).

The Stimulator

The stimulator generates a square wave electrical pulse that depolarizes the nerve under the cathode (i.e., the negative pole). This generates an action potential in the nerve that propagates up and down the nerve. The stimulator is synchronized with the oscilloscope sweep, thus enabling the propagated potential to be recorded at a distance by the recording electrodes (see Fig. 1-1).

The controls on the stimulator are used for adjusting the following:

1. Stimulus duration, which can be varied from 0.05 msec to 1.0 msec
2. Stimulus intensity, which can be increased in volts in a constant voltage stimulator or in milliamperes in a constant current stimulator
3. Rate of stimulation, which can be varied from 0.2 to 50 per second
4. Duration of a train during repetitive stimulation studies

For most nerve conduction studies (see Appendix I) a 0.1 to 0.2 msec pulse at a slow repetitive stimulation rate of 1 to 2 per second (Hz) is adequate. The intensity is gradually increased to get the maximal response and then a further 20 to 30 percent. This supramaximal test stimulus ensures activation of all the nerve fibers. Long duration and high intensity stimulation, besides being more uncomfortable for the patient, increases the stimulus artifact and may unintentionally stimulate adjacent nerves.

The *stimulus artifact* is the deflection from the baseline resulting from direct conduction of the stimulus. It is sometimes used for latency measurements as a marker of the onset of a sweep (see Figs. 1-8, 1-13).

At times, the stimulus artifact may be so large that it masks the onset of the response. This phenomenon results from the excessive cutaneous spread of the stimulating current to the recording electrodes and is particularly noticeable during sensory nerve conduction studies where higher amplification settings are used. The stimulus artifact can be reduced by:

1. Placing the ground between the stimulating and recording electrodes.
2. Adequate separation of stimulating, ground, and recording wires.
3. Ensuring equal impedance in both recording electrodes so that similar voltages are picked up by both the electrodes and suppressed by the differential amplifier.
4. Cleaning of any perspiration or conducting gel between the electrodes with alcohol or acetone to prevent the surface spread of stimulus.
5. Using the lowest stimulus intensity and duration necessary to get a supramaximal response. Rotating the anode of the stimulator is sometimes helpful.
6. Avoiding very short (<10 cm) distances between the stimulating and recording electrodes.
7. Using a higher value of low frequency filter helps early recovery of the artifact to baseline; using a lower value of high frequency filter can help to reduce the amplitude of the artifact.

Amplification and Filters
The very small potentials at the recording electrodes (microvolts for sensory potentials and millivolts for motor responses) have to be amplified up to a million times before they can be displayed. Differential amplifiers, which amplify the voltage difference between the active and reference recording electrodes, are used to amplify the signal. Unwanted interference signals are of equal voltage at both electrodes and therefore cancel out (this result is called common mode rejection).

Amplification settings determine the amplitude per division on the display screen. A sensitivity range of 0.5 μV per division to 10 mV per division can be selected depending on the expected amplitude of the response (see Appendix I).

FILTERS. Filters serve to reduce unwanted interference outside the frequency bandwidth of the electrical signals of interest.

The *high-frequency filter* attenuates the amplitude of high-frequency signals by 30 percent at the selected setting (cut-off frequency) and more for higher-frequency signals [11]. High-frequency background noise is filtered out with lower high-frequency filter settings during sensory studies (see Appendix I).

The *low-frequency filter* attenuates amplitudes of low-frequency signals by 30 percent at the selected setting (cut-off frequency) and more for lower-frequency signals [11]. Very low settings result in an unstable baseline.

Appropriate filter settings for different studies are listed in Appendix I. The use of incorrect filter settings can significantly affect amplitudes and, to a lesser extent, the latencies of the responses.

THE LOUDSPEAKER. Audio amplification during the needle examination helps in the recognition of many potentials by their characteristic sounds. During nerve conduction studies the stimuli can be heard as they are delivered. Auditory feedback of muscle activity can be used to help patients relax and is particularly useful during the sensory studies.

Display Screen (Cathode Ray Oscilloscope)
After amplification the potentials are displayed on a screen. Each trace displays the potentials picked up by one pair of recording electrodes, and most machines have at least two available channels. A timeline is displayed as a separate trace. The horizontal sweep speed of the trace can be selected from 0.2 to 500 msec/cm. For most routine nerve conduction studies sweep speeds betweeen 1 and 10 msec/cm are selected (see Appendix I) depending on the expected latency of the response.

During nerve conduction studies the stimulus triggers the oscilloscope sweep. During electromyography (EMG) the sweep can either run freely (restarting after reaching the end of the screen) or be triggered by a motor unit. The motor unit potential prior to the triggering point can be seen by setting a delay time. The potentials seen with each sweep are automatically erased with each new sweep although they can be recorded on paper or taped simultaneously. Digitized storage permits the potentials to be displayed on the screen until they are erased.

DIGITAL SIGNAL AVERAGER. The averager improves signal-to-noise ratio and is primarily used to obtain records of small amplitude sensory potentials free of background electrical noise. The signal, which is time-locked to the stimulus, averages at a constant latency, whereas the elec-

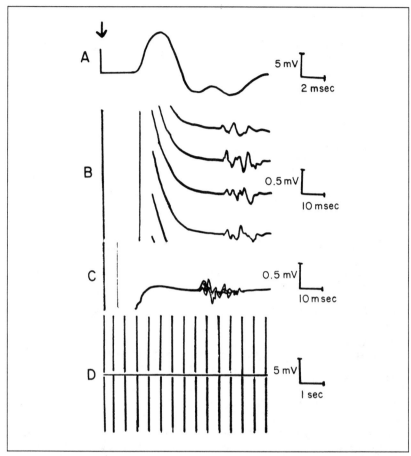

Figure 1-4. *Illustration of different recording modes. Arrow indicates the point of stimulation. A. Single sweep recording of a motor response. B. Raster recording of F-waves where successive sweeps are recorded in series. C. Superimposed F-waves. D. Continuous-mode recording of motor responses during 3-Hz repetitive stimulation. The time axis in the continuous mode is determined by the paper speed selected.*

trical noise, which occurs randomly, cancels out. The analog signals from the amplifier output are digitized (analog to digital conversion) prior to averaging. The analysis time (the sweep duration following the stimulus) and the number of trials to be averaged may need to be set on the averager controls before starting the averager.

Recording Apparatus
The displayed signals are recorded on paper, photographed, or tape-recorded on magnetic tape. Different modes may be available for recording on paper such as single sweep, superimposed, raster (sequential), and continuous (Fig. 1-4).

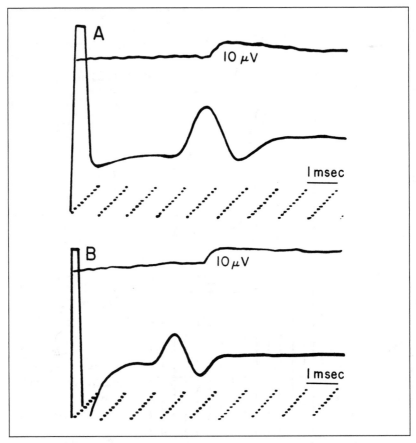

Figure 1-5. *Effect of temperature on a sural sensory nerve conduction study. A. Skin temperature = 29°C. B. Skin temperature = 34°C. Note the increased latency and amplitude at the lower recording temperature in* A.

The Skin Temperature Controlling Unit
The skin temperature controlling unit is an important accessory that uses an infrared heat lamp and a skin temperature sensor to increase the surface temperature to a preset level (usually 34°C). The recorded responses have an increased latency and amplitude and a reduced conduction velocity with low recording temperatures (Fig. 1-5). The skin temperature is recorded with a plate thermistor and appropriate corrections are made if necessary, as described later in this chapter.

Nerve Conduction Studies
General Considerations
Routine nerve conduction studies evaluate only large myelinated nerve fiber function. Electrophysiologic studies objectively document the pres-

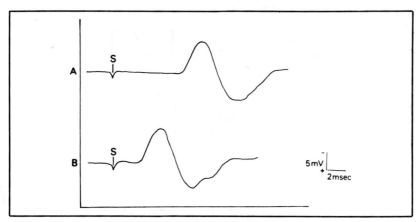

Figure 1-6. *Compound motor action potential (CMAP) from the abductor pollicis brevis following stimulation of the median nerve in the antecubital fossa* (A) *and at the wrist* (B).

ence and severity of any peripheral nerve dysfunction; its precise localization (neuronal cell body, roots, plexus, or peripheral nerve); its distribution (focal, multifocal, or diffuse); and the pathophysiology (segmental demyelination versus axonal degeneration).

The information obtained narrows the differential diagnosis and helps to plan treatment and determine prognosis. The electrophysiologic findings, however, are not pathognomonic of any specific disease, so their planning and meaningful interpretation requires clinical correlation.

Electrical stimulation of nerves initiates an action potential that travels in both directions from the point of stimulation.

By convention in neurophysiology, when the active recording electrode (G_1) is negative relative to the reference electrode (for example, when the wave of depolarization reaches the active electrode) the recorded potential has an upward deflection.

Motor Nerve Conduction Study
The motor nerve conduction study involves stimulating with supramaximal intensity (20 to 30 percent above stimulus intensity required to elicit a maximal response) an accessible motor or mixed nerve at two or more points along its course (Fig. 1-6). The motor response is recorded from a distal muscle innervated by the tested nerve employing the belly-tendon method (see Fig. 1-3C). This involves placing the active recording electrode (G_1; black) on the midpoint of the muscle belly (where the nerve endings terminate on the muscle) and the reference electrode (G_2; white) on the tendon. With this arrangement the recorded response is a biphasic potential with an initial larger upward (negative) deflection followed by a smaller downward (positive) deflection (Fig. 1-6). The

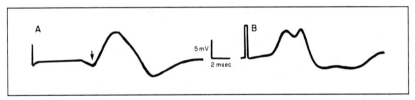

Figure 1-7. A. *An initial positivity* (arrow) *of the motor response is recorded when the active recording electrode is not directly over the motor point.* B. *Notched motor response is seen when the active recording electrode is placed between the motor points of two adjacent muscles.*

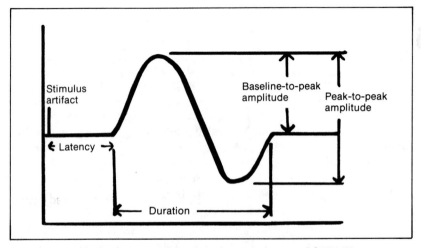

Figure 1-8. *Measured parameters of a compound motor action potential (CMAP).*

evoked motor response is called a compound muscle action potential (CMAP) because it is the sum of the action potentials of the individual muscle fibers. It is also referred to as the M-wave ("M" standing for motor).

If an initial positivity precedes the negative peak (Fig. 1-7A) then the following should be considered:

1. The active recording electrode is not over the endplate region.
2. The active and reference electrodes have been transposed.
3. Stimulation of neighboring nerves has occurred either by incorrect placement of stimulating electrodes or by spread of stimulus due to a high intensity of stimulus. The initial positivity in this instance is a result of the recording electrodes picking up a volume-conducted response from adjoining muscles.
4. There is an anomalous innervation.

A notched motor response (Fig. 1-7B) is seen when the active re-

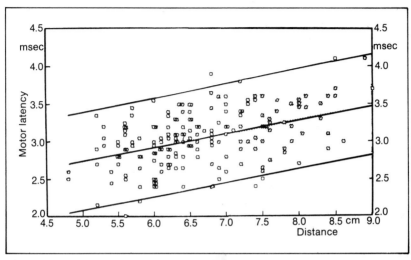

Figure 1-9. *Linear increase in the median nerve terminal motor latency with increasing distance from wrist to abductor pollicis brevis. The hatched area indicates the 95% confidence range. (From F. Bucthal, A. Rosenfalck, and W. Trojaborg. Electrophysiological findings in entrapment of median nerve in wrist and elbow.* J. Neurol. Neurosurg. Psychiatry 37:340, 1974. *Used by permission.)*

cording electrode is placed between the recording points of two adjacent muscles.

The latency, amplitude, and duration are measured as shown in Figure 1-8. The distance between the center of the cathode and the center of the active recording electrode (G_1) is measured in millimeters using a flexible tape. An obstetric caliper is used for distance measurements when the path of the nerve is nonlinear.

The *motor latency* is the time interval between the onset of the stimulus and the initial deflection of the motor response (Fig. 1-8) measured in milliseconds (10^{-3} seconds). It includes not only the nerve conduction time in the motor fibers but also the neuromuscular transmission time, which precludes the calculation of the conduction velocity in the distal segment.

The *distal motor latency* obtained by stimulation at the most distal site along the nerve reflects conduction time in the most distal segment.

Latency measurements are an important cause of nonphysiologic errors, so it is important to observe the following technical details meticulously:

1. Standard distances between the most distal stimulating site and the active recording electrode enable meaningful interpretation of distal latency measurements, since the latency is directly proportional to the distance (Fig. 1-9). The recommended standard distance for the median

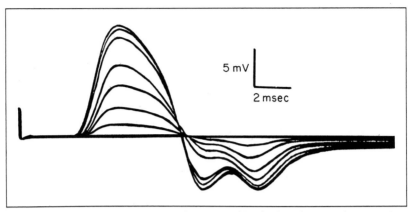

Figure 1-10. *Median motor responses with increasing stimulus intensity. Note the progressive decline in latency with increasing stimulus intensity.*

nerve is 6.5 cm, ulnar nerve 7 cm, peroneal nerve 9 cm, and tibial nerve 10 cm [14]. If a standard distance is not used, a correction for the standard distance can be made using the following formula [14]:

$$\text{Latency correction (msec)} = \frac{\text{measured-standard distance (mm)}}{\text{conduction velocity (m/sec)}}$$

For example: Median nerve stimulation from wrist to abductor pollicis brevis

Standard distance	= 65 mm
Distance used	= 85 mm
Median nerve conduction velocity	= 50 m/sec

$$\text{Latency correction (msec) to standard distance} = \frac{85 \text{ mm} - 65 \text{ mm}}{50 \text{ m/sec}} = 0.4 \text{ msec}$$

In this example if the latency obtained with a distance of 85 mm was 4.2 msec, then the latency corrected to the standard distance of 65 mm would be 4.2 msec − 0.4 msec = 3.8 msec.

2. The stimulus intensity should always be supramaximal to ensure stimulation of all the nerve fascicles. There is a progressive decrease in latency with an increase in stimulus intensity from submaximal to supramaximal (Fig. 1-10). This decrease in latency is due to the spread of stimulus distal to the point of stimulation [3,5,8,12,13,16].

3. It is often difficult to decide the exact point for latency measurement with the lower gain settings used for amplitude measurement because the baseline deflection is not sharp (Fig. 1-11). This results in a tendency for longer latency to be reported [5]. Amplification of the response by

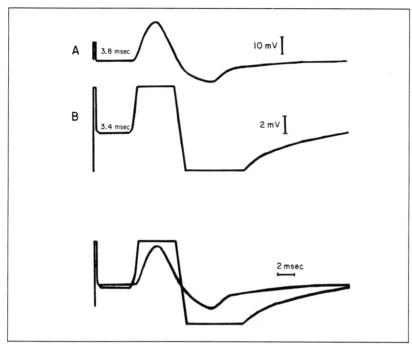

Figure 1-11. *Median motor responses at amplification settings of 10 mV/cm* (A) *and 2 mV/cm* (B). *The sharper and more clearly defined take-off with the higher amplification setting results in a shorter latency measurement* (B).

using a higher sensitivity setting by a factor of 4 to 5 results in a sharper takeoff and a more clearly defined onset for latency measurements (Fig. 1-11).

The *conduction velocity (CV)* in motor fibers is calculated indirectly:

$$CV \text{ (m/sec)} = \frac{\text{distance (mm) between proximal and distal stimulating sites}}{\text{proximal latency (msec)} - \text{distal latency (msec)}}$$

For example: Distance between proximal and distal stimulating sites = 200 mm

Proximal latency = 6 msec

Distal latency = 3 msec

$$CV = \frac{200 \text{ mm}}{6 \text{ msec} - 3 \text{ msec}} = \frac{200 \text{ mm}}{3 \text{ msec}} = 66.7 \text{ m/sec}$$

The latency (measured to the onset of the CMAP) and the conduction velocity represent conduction in the large diameter, fastest conducting fibers. It follows, therefore, that if a few fast conducting fibers are spared in a peripheral nerve lesion, the latency and conduction velocity could remain normal. The range of conduction velocities of individual nerve fibers within the peripheral nerves measured by collision techniques does not generally exceed 40 percent. In peripheral neuropathies with pure axonal degenerations the conduction velocity is reduced by less than 40 percent of the mean [6]. Conversely, in segmental demyelination, which impairs saltatory conduction in myelinated nerve fibers, the conduction velocity is often slowed by greater than 40 percent of the normal mean [6,7,9].

Amplitude measurements (see Fig. 1-8) are made from baseline to peak or from negative to positive peak (peak to peak) and are expressed in millivolts (10^{-3} V). The amplitude determination is an estimation of the number of muscle fibers activated by the nerve stimulation and represents the sum of the amplitudes of the individual muscle fibers underlying the active recording electrode. A reduced motor amplitude can result from disorders of the muscle, neuromuscular junction (e.g., myasthenic syndrome), or peripheral nerve. In peripheral nerve lesions with axonal loss the amplitude may be normal, if adequate reinnervation has occurred. A sudden change in amplitude with proximal stimulation can be due to conduction block (see Fig. 20-1) and is useful for localizing focal nerve lesions. Motor response amplitude is an insensitive measure of mild neurogenic lesions because of the wide variation in normal subjects.

Duration and shape reflect the synchrony of contraction of the muscle fibers contributing to the response and indirectly to the uniformity of conduction velocities of the stimulated nerve fibers. The duration is generally longer with more proximal stimulation because the range of conduction time among the individual fibers increases with longer distances. *Dispersion* of the compound motor action potential (see Fig. 20-5) is an increase in the duration and number of turns (spikes without baseline crossings) or phases (spikes with baseline crossings). Dispersion occurs when some axons conduct slowly (e.g., acute demyelinating diseases).

Sensory Nerve Conduction Study
Sensory potentials (Fig. 1-12) are unaffected by lesions proximal to the dorsal root ganglion (cell body of the sensory fibers) in spite of sensory loss. They are therefore useful in localizing a lesion either proximal (root or spinal cord) or distal (plexus or nerve) to the dorsal root ganglia.

Sensory nerve conduction studies are more sensitive than motor nerve conduction studies for detecting mild peripheral nerve dysfunction. Sensory responses are more difficult to record because of their small size, so greater attention to technical detail as well as signal averaging is often necessary to obtain a clean recording. The high amplification setting (5 to 10 μV/cm) required also increases the size of the stimulus artifact.

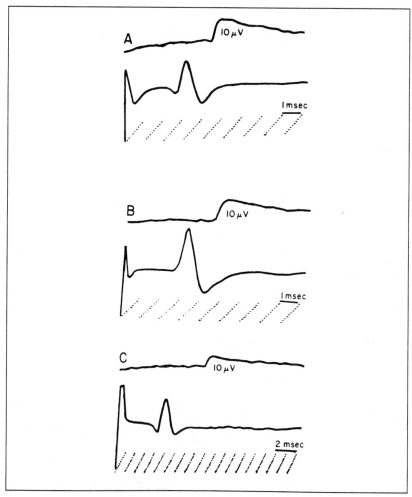

Figure 1-12. *Normal median sensory responses recorded 14 cm from the stimulating electrode. A. Orthodromic. B. Antidromic. Note the latencies are identical but the antidromic amplitude is larger due to the closer proximity of digital nerves to the recording electrodes. Median mixed nerve action potential recorded at the elbow with wrist stimulation* (C).

Background muscle activity is often picked up at these amplifications but can be reduced by providing the patient with auditory feedback while he or she tries to relax the muscles. Electrical noise frequently distorts the waveform and can be reduced by disconnecting any unnecessary nearby cables and switching off fluorescent lighting.

A supramaximal stimulus can be delivered distally to the digital sensory nerves using ring electrodes or proximally over the nerve trunk with the cathode placed closer to the active recording electrode (G_1).

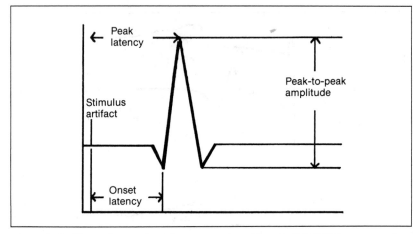

Figure 1-13. *Measured parameters of a sensory nerve action potential (SNAP).*

The action potential travels in both directions from the point of stimulation. The recording electrodes are placed 3 to 4 cm apart with the active recording electrode (G_1; black) placed at a distance of 10 to 15 cm from the cathode (see Fig. 1-3). Larger distances tend to increase dispersion and decrease the already small amplitude of the sensory response.

Recording of sensory responses can be *orthodromic* (toward the spinal cord in the direction of physiologic conduction) with digital nerve stimulation or *antidromic* (direction opposite to physiologic conduction) with proximal stimulation of the nerve trunk (see Figs. 1-3, 1-12). The speed of conduction is the same in orthodromic and antidromic recordings (Fig. 1-12). The amplitude of antidromic sensory responses is larger with surface electrode recording because of the closer proximity of the digital nerves to the recording electrode (Fig. 1-12). An antidromic recording from mixed nerve stimulation is often followed by a motor response that may distort the small sensory response. Muscle artifact does not occur with stimulation of sensory nerves like the sural, superficial radial, and superficial peroneal, for which antidromic recording is preferred.

An orthodromically recorded response is typically a triphasic wave (Fig. 1-13) with an initial small downward deflection (positivity) due to current flow from the potential as it approaches the active recording electrode. This is followed by a large upward deflection (negativity) resulting from depolarization under the active electrode and finally by a small late positivity due to current flow of the potential moving away from the active recording electrode [8]. Antidromically recorded sensory responses are usually biphasic with an initial large upward deflection (negativity) followed by a small downward deflection (positivity) (see Fig. 1-12).

The sensory response is called the sensory compound nerve action potential (CNAP) since it represents the sum of the action potentials of the individual nerve fibers. The latency and amplitude are the important measured parameters of the sensory CNAP (Fig. 1-13). The distance is measured in millimeters from the center of the cathode to the center of the active recording electrode using a flexible tape.

The *sensory latency* is measured in milliseconds from the stimulus onset to the initial positive peak, or the beginning of the subsequent negative deflection if a preceding positive peak is not recorded (Fig. 1-13). This onset latency represents conduction in the fastest nerve fibers.

The peak latency is measured from the stimulus onset to the negative peak (Fig. 1-13), and is particularly useful when the onset is not sharp or is obscured by stimulus artifact. The peak latency is at least 0.4 msec longer than onset latency, and the conduction velocity calculated from peak latency is 5 to 10 m/sec slower [11].

Meaningful comparisons of the sensory latency require strict standardization of distance, which is not always practical.

The *conduction velocity* (m/sec) is calculated by dividing the conduction distance in millimeters by the sensory latency in milliseconds. It is preferred to the latency as a parameter of sensory conduction time since it does not require standardization of distance.

The *amplitude* is measured from peak to peak (Fig. 1-13) in microvolts (10^{-6} V). The amplitude is an estimation of the number of nerve fibers activated but is heavily influenced by the distance between the nerve and the recording electrode. The rise time (onset to the peak of the negative deflection) is prolonged when the amplitude is reduced as a result of an increase in distance between the nerve and the recording electrode.

Mixed Nerve Conduction Studies

Median, ulnar, and peroneal nerves are stimulated distally over the nerve trunks and potentials are recorded proximally over the respective nerves (see Fig. 1-12C). Mixed nerve conduction studies are principally used in trying to localize more proximal lesions because sensory potentials are often too small to be picked up consistently at the proximal sites. The large diameter sensory fibers have a lower threshold and conduct faster than motor fibers by about 5 to 10 percent [3]. Mixed nerve conduction time pertains to the sensory fibers in normal nerves but not in patients with peripheral nerve disease where there is early involvement of the sensory fibers [2,8]. The technical details of recording are similar to the orthodromic sensory studies.

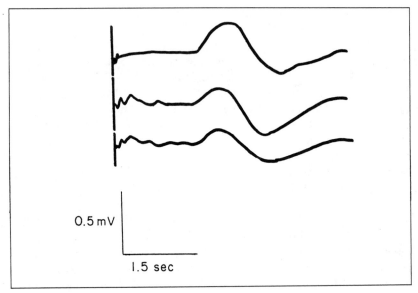

Figure 1-14. *Sympathetic skin response.*

Sympathetic Skin Response

The high threshold for electric stimulation precludes direct evaluation of the small unmyelinated nerve fibers. The exact mechanism of generation of the sympathetic skin response (SSR) and the central pathways involved are uncertain. The activity in the sweat glands (sudomotor activity) is regulated by the sympathetic nervous system. The SSR is the electrodermal activity caused by alterations in the electrical skin resistance from minute changes in the sudomotor activity and serves as an indirect assessment of the autonomic nervous system [15]. A variety of sensory stimuli (auditory, tactile, and deep inspiration) can elicit an SSR.

The active (G_1) recording electrode is commonly placed over the palm of the hand or the plantar surface of the foot and the corresponding reference electrode is placed on the dorsum of the hand or foot, but proximal recording sites can also be used [15]. Electrical stimuli, 0.1 to 0.2 msec in duration and 10 to 20 mA in intensity, can be applied to the digits, wrist, or ankle on either side to depolarize the sensory nerves. Habituation of the response is common, so a random stimulation frequency is preferable. A band pass of 0.5 Hz to 2 kHz is optimum for recording the low frequencies in the potentials. The recorded response may have one to three phases (Fig. 1-14). The latency is not useful clinically and is mainly affected by the height of the subject and the position of the recording electrodes. Since the unmyelinated sympathetic fibers conduct at 1 to 2 m/sec, the expected latency is about 1.5 seconds in the hand and close to 2 seconds in the foot. The peak-to-peak am-

Table 1-1. *Mean Motor Nerve Conduction Velocities at Different Ages*

Average age of group (weeks)	Ulnar (m/sec)	Median (m/sec)	Peroneal (m/sec)	Posterior tibial (m/sec)
5	34.5	33.1	37.2	34.3
18	35.4	35.8	39.1	32.7
34	46.1	41.8	44.1	38.3
56	46.7	40.4	46.7	39.8
88	51.6	47.5	49.5	44.5
140	52.4	49.4	44.2	43.1
210	56.1	54.9	52.2	48.4

Source: Adapted from R. D. Baer and E. W. Johnson. Motor nerve conduction velocities in normal children. *Arch. Phys. Med. Rehabil.* October: 698, 1965. Used by permission.

plitude is 0.5 to 3.0 mV. Appendix I lists the appropriate machine settings. *The sympathetic skin response (SSR) is normal when present and abnormal when absent.* An absent SSR in patients with neuropathies correlates with involvement of unmyelinated autonomic fibers [15].

Normal Values
The normal values for most of the commonly used nerves are tabulated in Appendixes II and III and in the sections on individual nerves that follow. Because techniques differ between laboratories, databases to define criteria of abnormality should be established in each laboratory. The nerve conduction velocity and latency values of nerves show a bell-shaped gaussian distribution in the normal population, therefore, most laboratories use two standard deviations from the mean as the normal range. However, amplitude measurements are more variable and the distribution does not follow a gaussian curve, so the lowest value in the range from normal controls is often used. The latencies and conduction velocities with *near nerve recordings* are comparable to those with surface recordings, but the amplitudes are about three times higher since the recording electrode is very close to the nerve.

Physiologic Variations in Normal Values
AGE. Nerve conduction velocities at birth are about 50 percent of adult values and even slower in premature infants, increasing rapidly to about 75 percent by 12 months and 100 percent by about 4 to 5 years (Table 1-1). Myelination and increase in size of fibers is usually complete by 5 years. Appendix III gives the conduction velocities of commonly tested nerves in children. There is gradual slowing of conduction velocities and reduction in amplitudes of motor and sensory responses from the second

decade onward and the decline gets slightly steeper after the sixth decade [14]. In general, the decline is about 3 percent per decade after 30 years [1].

TEMPERATURE. There is a progressive increase in latency and a decrease in conduction velocity with decreasing temperature [4] (see Fig. 1-5). If the surface temperature is below 34°C, a correction of 2 m/sec should be added to the calculated conduction velocity and 0.2 msec subtracted from the measured latency for each degree Celsius below 34 [1]. However, it is preferable to warm the extremities prior to the conduction study since the use of corrections tends to introduce additional errors.

VARIATION IN DIFFERENT NERVES AND SEGMENTS. Upper extremity nerve conduction velocities are generally 10 to 15 percent faster than those of the lower extremity. The lower limit of conduction velocity is generally around 50 m/sec in the upper extremities and about 45 m/sec for the lower extremities, except the sural nerve where it is 40 m/sec.

Conduction velocity in the proximal nerve segments is generally 5 to 10 percent faster than in the distal segments. These variations may be due to lower temperatures and smaller size of nerve fibers distally [1].

Sensory conduction time is generally about 5 percent faster than motor, but the conduction velocity in motor and sensory fibers varies randomly in practice because of normal errors in distance calculation [1].

Orthodromic conduction velocity is the same as antidromic, but the amplitudes are larger with antidromic surface recordings because of the closer proximity of the digital nerves to the recording electrode.

Experimental Errors in Nerve Conduction Studies
Even in technically perfect recordings there can be an error of 5 to 10 percent, most of which is due to observer errors in distance and time measurements [10].

References
1. Bucthal, F., and Rosenfalck, A. Evoked action potentials and conduction velocity in human sensory nerves. *Brain Res.* 3:1, 1966.
2. Bucthal, F., Rosenfalck, A., and Trojaborg, W. Electrophysiological findings in entrapment of the median nerve at wrist and elbow. *J. Neurol. Neurosurg. Psychiatry* 37:340, 1974.
3. Dawson, G. D. The relative excitability of conduction velocity of sensory and motor fibers in man. *J. Physiol.* 131:436, 1956.
4. Denys, E. H. *Minimonograph #14: The role of temperature in electromyography*. Rochester, Minnesota: American Association of Electromyography and Electrodiagnosis, 1980.

5. Gassel, M. M.   Source of error in motor nerve conduction studies. *Neurology (Minneap.)* 14:825, 1964.
6. Gilliat, R. W.   Nerve conduction in human and experimental neuropathies. *Proc. R. Soc. Med.* 59:989, 1966.
7. Gilliat, R. W.   Recent advances in the pathophysiology of nerve conduction. In J. E. Desmedt (Ed.), *New Developments in EMG and Clinical Neurophysiology*, Vol. 2. Karger: Basel, 1973.
8. Gilliat, R. W., Melville, I. D., Velate, A. S., and Willison, R. G.   A study of normal nerve action potentials using an averaging technique (barrier grid storage tube). *J. Neurol. Neurosurg. Psychiatry* 28:191, 1965.
9. Mcleod, J. G., Prineas, J. W., and Walsh, J. C.   The relationship of conduction velocity to pathology in peripheral nerves: A study of sural nerve in 90 patients. In J. E. Desmedt (Ed.), *New developments in EMG and Clinical Neurophysiology*, Vol. 2. Karger: Basel, 1973.
10. Maynard, F. M., and Stolov, W. C.   Experimental error in determination of nerve conduction velocity. *Arch. Phy. Med. Rehabil.* 53:362, 1972.
11. Oh, S. H.   *Clinical Electromyography: Nerve Conduction Studies*. Baltimore: University Park Press, 1984.
12. Preswick, G.   The effect of stimulus intensity on motor latency in carpal tunnel syndrome. *J. Neurol. Neurosurg. Psychiatry* 26:398, 1963.
13. Pinelli, P.   Physical, anatomical and physiological factors in the latency measurement of the M response. *Electroenceph. Clin. Neurophysiol.* 17:86, 1964.
14. Rigshospitalet Laboratory of Clinical Neurophysiology. *Electromyography: Sensory and Motor Conduction. Findings in Normal Subjects*. Copenhagen: Rigshospitalet, 1975.
15. Shahani, B. T., Halperin, J. J., Boulu, P., and Cohen, J.   Sympathetic skin response: A method of assessing unmyelinated axon dysfunction in peripheral neuropathies. *J. Neurol. Neurosurg. Psychiatry* 47:536, 1984.
16. Wiederholt, W. C.   Threshold and conduction velocity in isolated mixed mammalian nerves. *Neurology (Minneap.)* 20:347, 1970.

Brachial Plexus 2
Motor Studies

Anatomy

The *brachial plexus* is composed of the ventral rami of $C_{5,6,7,8}$ and T_1 spinal nerves (Fig. 2-1). The five ventral rami merge into three trunks that pass as a compact bundle over the first rib and behind the middle third of the clavicle to enter the axilla. Each trunk divides into anterior and posterior divisions and then unite to form three cords (lateral, medial, and posterior) from which the peripheral nerves to the upper limb are formed.

Applications

Brachial plexus and cervical root stimulation are used to document impaired conduction in proximal neurogenic lesions involving the cervical roots, brachial plexus, or proximal nerve trunks. Latency measurements

Figure 2-1. *Simplified plan of brachial plexus emphasizing commonly studied nerves. (U,M,L = upper, middle, and lower trunks; A,P = anterior and posterior divisions of each trunk; lateral, medial, posterior cords.)*

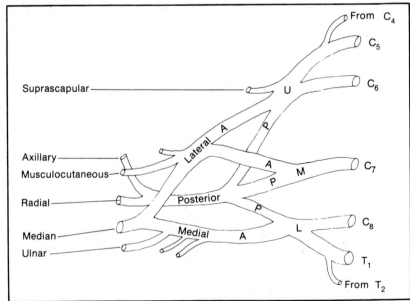

can clarify some of these problems [3]. In unilateral lesions a latency difference exceeding 1 msec between the left and right sides is probably more sensitive, provided the distances between the stimulating and recording electrodes are identical on both sides and a more distal lesion has been excluded [1,6]. The amplitudes are generally greater than 5 mV [7], but the marked variability with needle recordings makes them less useful in side-to-side comparisons.

Repetitive stimulation at Erb's point with recording from proximal muscles increases the diagnostic yield in myasthenia gravis.

Procedure

1. Recording electrode placement (Figs. 2-2 to 2-6). The muscles often used for recording are biceps ($C_{5,6}$ roots, lateral cord, musculocuta-

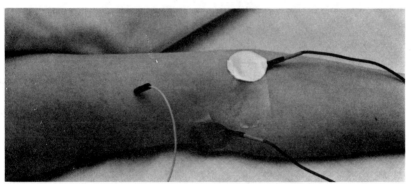

Figure 2-2. *Placement of recording electrodes for study of the biceps brachii.*

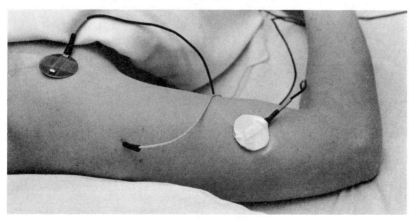

Figure 2-3. *Placement of recording electrodes for study of the deltoid.*

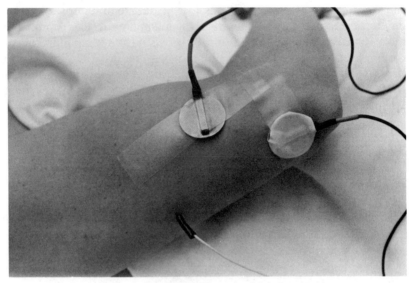

Figure 2-4. Placement of recording electrodes for study of the triceps.

neous nerve), deltoid ($C_{5,6}$ roots, posterior cord, circumflex nerve), triceps ($C_{6,7,8}$ roots, posterior cord, radial nerve), supraspinatus and infraspinatus ($C_{5,6}$ roots, suprascapular nerve), abductor digiti quinti (C_8,T_1 roots, medial cord, ulnar nerve), and abductor pollicis brevis (C_8,T_1 roots, medial cord, median nerve). *Surface electrodes* are used to record over the intrinsic hand muscles. Figure 2-7 illustrates a

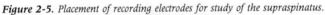

Figure 2-5. Placement of recording electrodes for study of the supraspinatus.

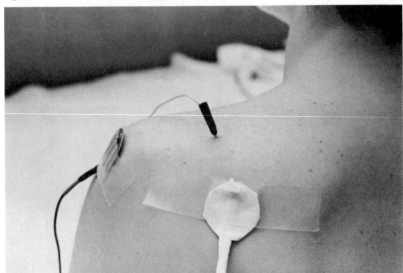

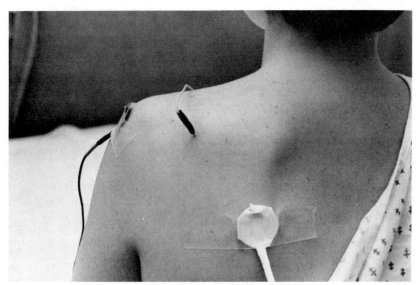

Figure 2-6. *Placement of recording electrodes for study of the infraspinatus.*

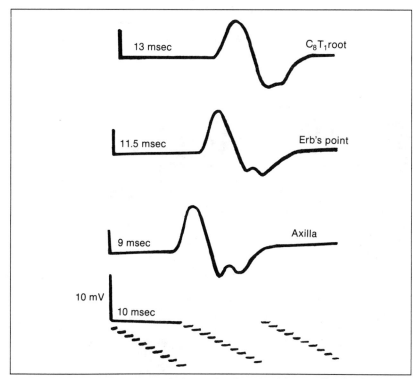

Figure 2-7. *Normal motor responses with recording from the abductor pollicis brevis on stimulation of the C_8–T_1 roots, Erb's point, and axilla.*

normal response with recording from the abductor pollicis brevis. *Needle recordings* are preferred for proximal muscles to avoid recording volume-conducted responses from adjoining muscles resulting from multiple nerves being stimulated. A concentric or monopolar needle electrode is placed in the appropriate muscle for recording.

    a. G_1 monopolar needle electrode is placed in the muscle to be tested.

    b. G_2 surface disc electrode is placed distal to G_1 over the tendon.

2. Ground is placed between the stimulating and recording electrodes.
3. Stimulation

    a. Surface stimulation at the axilla (Fig. 2-8) and Erb's point (Fig. 2-9)

    b. Monopolar needle stimulation of cervical roots (Fig. 2-10)

4. Distances from stimulating to recording electrodes around the shoulder are measured with calipers.

Brachial Plexus Stimulation

Erb's point, located just above the clavicle in the angle between the posterior edge of the sternomastoid muscle and the clavicle, is the most accessible site for stimulation of the trunks of the brachial plexus (see Fig. 2-9). Stimulation at Erb's point (Fig. 2-9) is generally uncomfortable for the patient. The deeper location of the nerves often necessitates higher intensity of stimulation to get a supramaximal response. Multiple nerves are stimulated simultaneously, resulting in jerking of the whole arm, which needs to be appropriately restrained to avoid injury and to

Figure 2-8. *Stimulation at axilla.*

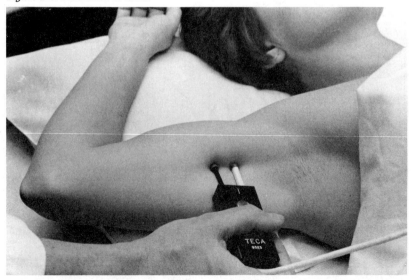

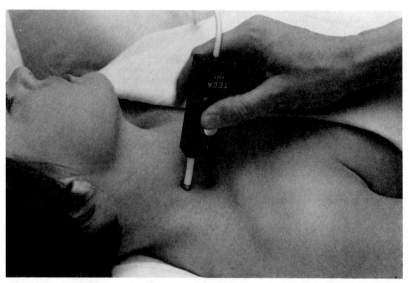

Figure 2-9. *Stimulation at Erb's point.*

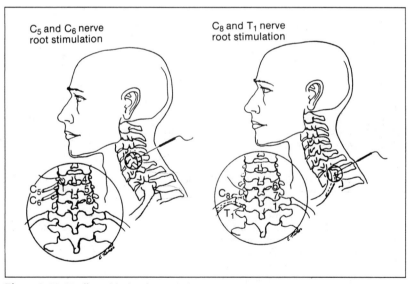

Figure 2-10. *Needle positioning for cervical root stimulation. (From: I. C. MacLean. Nerve root stimulation to evaluate conduction across the brachial and lumbosacral plexus.* Third Annual Continuing Education Course. *American Association of Electromyography and Electrodiagnosis, Philadelphia, PA, 1980. Used by permission.)*

prevent artifacts from movement. Table 2-1 lists brachial plexus latencies from Erb's point.

Cervical Root Stimulation

Cervical root stimulation in general is better tolerated. A 50 to 70 mm monopolar needle (cathode) is inserted perpendicular to the skin in the posterior paraspinal area until the tip is in contact with the transverse process (Fig. 2-10). Insertion 1 to 2 cm lateral to the C_5 spine stimulates the $C_{5,6}$ roots. The needle is placed about 1 cm caudal and lateral to the C_7 spinal process to stimulate the C_8,T_1 roots. Insertion of the needle between these two points is used to activate the $C_{6,7}$ roots. The anode

Table 2-1. *Brachial Plexus Latencies from Erb's Point*

Muscle	Distance from Erb's point (cm)	Latency (SD in msec)
Biceps brachii (Fig. 2-2)	20.0	4.6 ± 0.6
	24.0	4.7 ± 0.6
	28.0	5.0 ± 0.5
Deltoid (Fig. 2-3)	15.5	4.3 ± 0.5
	18.5	4.4 ± 0.35
Triceps brachii (Fig. 2-4)	21.5	4.5 ± 0.42
	26.5	4.9 ± 0.45
	31.5	5.3 ± 0.32
Supraspinatus (Fig. 2-5)	8.5	2.6 ± 0.32
	10.5	2.7 ± 0.27
Infraspinatus (Fig. 2-6)	14.0	3.4 ± 0.4
	17.0	3.4 ± 0.5

Source: Modified from Gassel [3].

Table 2-2. *Cervical Root Stimulation: Normal Values*

Segment	Latency (msec) mean ± SD	Conduction velocity (m/sec) mean ± SD	Reference
$C_{5,6}$–biceps	5.3 ± 0.4		[9]
C_{6-8}–triceps	5.4 ± 0.4		[9]
C_8, T_1–ADQ	13.5 ± 0.8 (12–14.5)		[10][a]
C_8–axilla (25 cm)	4.7 ± 0.5 (3.7–5.5)		[9]
C_8, T_1–axilla		76.1 ± 5.4	[8][b]
C_8, T_1–wrist		54.0 ± 2.4	[6]
R-L latency difference	<1 msec		[6,7,9]

ADQ = abductor digiti quinti.
[a] 10 patients (29–72 yr); C_8 = ADQ distance 70–81 cm; limb temperature 34°C at wrist.
[b] Percutaneous stimulation anterior to the C_7 transverse process.

Table 2-3. *Brachial Plexus Conduction Velocities*

Nerve	Erb's point–axilla mean ± SD (m/sec)	Normal limit (m/sec)	Reference
Musculocutaneous	58.0 ± 4.0	50	[11]
Axillary	62.2 ± 6.8	50	[2]
Radial	74.0 ± 6.7	61	[4]
Median	65.1 ± 6.1	53	[5]
R-L difference	—	14	[5]
Ulnar	63.0 ± 5.5	52	[5]
R-L difference	—	12	[5]

is a metal disc or plate and is placed slightly lateral to the monopolar needle electrode or on the anterior neck. Placing the anode medial and 1 cm caudal to the cathode is thought to stimulate the roots more proximally [1]. The responses are recorded from the appropriate root-innervated muscles (Table 2-2).

Axillary Stimulation
Axillary stimulation is done with bipolar surface electrodes over the axillary artery, in the groove between the corachobrachialis muscle anteriorly and the triceps posteriorly. It serves to compute a conduction velocity across the brachial plexus (Erb's point-axilla segment, Table 2-3).

References
1. Berger, A. R., Busis, N. A., Logigian, E. L., et al. Cervical root stimulation in the diagnosis of radiculopathy. *Neurology (Minneap.)* 37:329, 1987.
2. Currier, D. P. Motor conduction velocity of axillary nerve. *Phys. Ther.* 51:503, 1971.
3. Gassel, M. M. A test of nerve conduction to the muscles of the shoulder girdle in the diagnosis of proximal neurogenic and muscular disease. *J. Neurol. Neurosurg. Psychiatry* 27:200, 1964.
4. Gassel, M. M., and Diamantopoulos, E. Pattern of conduction times in the distribution of the radial nerve: A clinical and electrophysiologic study. *Neurology (Minneap.)* 14:222, 1964.
5. Ginzberg, M., Lee, M., Ginzburg, J., et al. Median and ulnar nerve conduction determinations in the Erb's point-axilla segment in normal subjects. *J. Neurol. Neurosurg. Psychiatry* 41:444, 1978.
6. Johnson, E. W. Spinal nerve stimulation. Thirty-third Annual Meeting, Didactic Program, American Association of Electromyography and Electrodiagnosis, September 1986, Boston, MA.
7. Kraft, G. H., and Johnson, E. W. Proximal motor nerve conduction and late responses: An AAEE workshop. American Association of Electromyography and Electrodiagnosis, September 1986, Boston, MA.
8. Krogness, K. Ulnar trunk conduction studies in the diagnosis of the thoracic outlet syndrome. *Acta Chir. Scand.* 129:597, 1973.

9. MacLean, I. C.   Nerve root stimulation to evaluate conduction across the brachial and lumbosacral plexuses. Third Annual Continuing Education Course, American Association of Electromyography and Electrodiagnosis, September 1980, Philadelphia, PA.
10. Sethi, R. K., and Krarup, C. C_8,T_1 root stimulation. (Unpublished data).
11. Trojaborg, W.   Motor and sensory conduction in the musculocutaneous nerve. *J. Neurol. Neurosurg. Psychiatry* 32:354, 1976.

Ulnar Nerve 3
Motor and Sensory Studies

Anatomy

The *ulnar nerve* is derived from the C_8 and T_1 roots, lower trunk, and medial cord of the brachial plexus. It is palpable behind the medial epicondyle in the *ulnar sulcus* after which it descends for about 1.5 to 4.0 cm [9] and then passes between the aponeurotic origin of the two heads of the flexor carpi ulnaris (*cubital tunnel*) to course deep in the forearm. At the wrist it is again superficial, lying just radial to the flexor carpi ulnaris tendon. The *dorsal sensory branch*, which provides sensory innervation to the ulnar part of the back of the hand and parts of the dorsum of the little and ring fingers, leaves the ulnar nerve about 5 to 8 cm proximal to the ulnar styloid process. The ulnar nerve enters the hand by passing through the *canal of Guyon*, formed by the pisiform bone and the hook of the hamate, and immediately divides into a superficial sensory and a deep motor branch. The ulnar nerve provides motor innervation to the flexor carpi ulnaris, to the ulnar half of the flexor digitorum profundus in the forearm, and to the hypothenar eminence muscles, adductor pollicis, interossei and ulnar lumbricals in the hand. The sensory innervation is to the skin of the ulnar aspect of the hand, the fifth digit, and the ulnar half of the fourth digit (Fig. 3-1).

Applications

Ulnar nerve entrapment at the elbow is the second most common upper extremity compression neuropathy and occurs either at the level of the ulnar sulcus or 1.5 to 4.0 cm below the ulnar sulcus between the two heads of the flexor carpi ulnaris (cubital tunnel syndrome) [9]. Less frequently, it is involved in compressive lesions in the hand, wrist (Guyon's canal), and thoracic outlet. Transsulcal slowing of greater than 10 m/sec is useful for localization of the lesion to the elbow region but should not be used as the only criterion of abnormality [2,12,13].

Procedure

Motor

1. Recording electrode placement (Fig. 3-2).
   a. G_1 is placed over the midportion of the abductor digiti quinti.
   b. G_2 is placed over the proximal phalanx of the fifth digit.

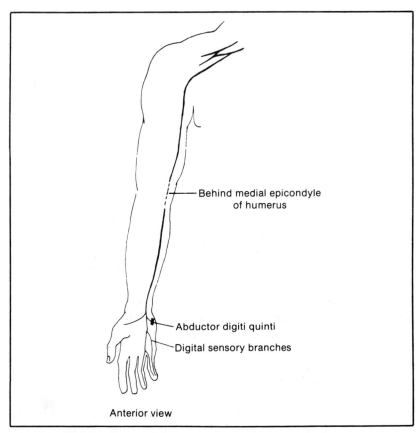

Behind medial epicondyle
of humerus

Abductor digiti quinti

Digital sensory branches

Anterior view

Figure 3-1. *Origin and course of ulnar nerve.*

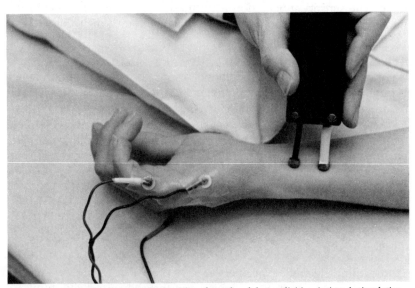

Figure 3-2. *Electrode placement for recording from the abductor digiti quinti and stimulation of ulnar nerve at the wrist.*

32

2. Ground is placed over the dorsum of the hand (Fig. 3-3).
3. Stimulation
   a. Palmar aspect of wrist just radial to the flexor carpi ulnaris tendon with the cathode 7 cm proximal to G_1 (Fig. 3-2).
   b. 3 to 5 cm distal to the ulnar sulcus (osseous groove in the posterior aspect of the medial epicondyle of the humerus) (Fig. 3-4).

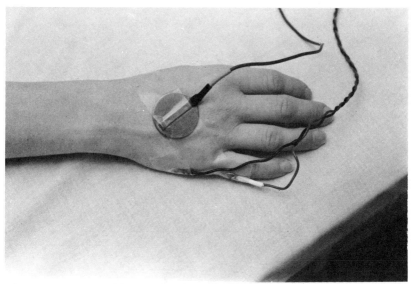

Figure 3-3. *Placement of the ground on the dorsum of the hand.*

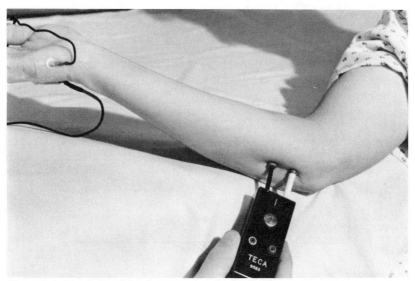

Figure 3-4. *Stimulation of the ulnar nerve just distal to the ulnar groove.*

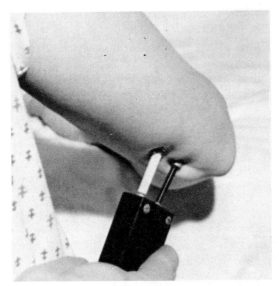

Figure 3-5. *Stimulation of the ulnar nerve just proximal to the ulnar groove.*

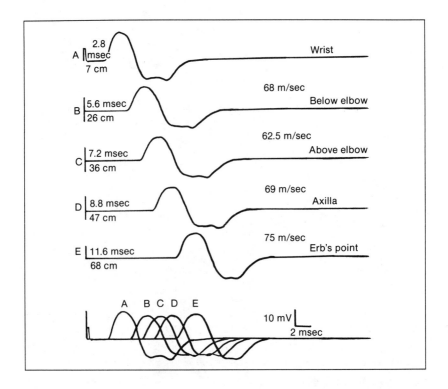

c. 5 to 7 cm proximal to the ulnar sulcus (Fig. 3-5). The distance between stimulation points across the elbow should be about 10 cm.
d. Axilla (see Fig. 2-8).
e. Erb's point (see Fig. 2-9).

Figure 3-6 shows a normal motor response from these stimulation sites. Normal values are listed in Table 3-1.

Table 3-1. Normal Values: Ulnar Motor

Segment	Distant latency or NCV	Amplitude (mV) peak to peak	Reference
Wrist to ADQ		12.2 ± 3.5 (>5.0) mV	[7]
Wrist to ADQ (distance 7 cm)	2.5 ± 0.25 (1.9–3.0 msec)		[13]
R-L difference (ADQ)	(<1.0) msec		[6]
Wrist to FDI	3.5 ± 0.36 (2.8–4.2) msec	>6 mV	[7,11]
R-L difference (FDI)	<1.3 msec		[11]
Latency difference FDI–ADQ	<2.0 msec		[11,12]
Wrist to flexor carpi ulnaris*			
(10 cm)	(2.1–3.4) msec	6–33 mV	[13]
(14 cm)	(2.7–3.9) msec		
Below elbow to wrist	62.5 ± 6.3 (51–73) m/sec		[7]
Above elbow to wrist	59.8 ± 5.0 (50.6–67.9)		[7]
Across elbow			[7]
70° (flexion)	59.7 ± 4.6 (50.8–68.4) m/sec		
180° (straight)	53.1 ± 4.0 (44.0–58.3) m/sec		
Axilla to above elbow	64.5 ± 5.1 (56.0–73.5) m/sec		[7]
Erb's point to axilla	63.0 ± 5.5 (55.0–73.2) m/sec		[3]
Erb's point to above elbow	61.3 ± 5.4 (52.0–78.0) m/sec		[5]

ADQ = abductor digiti quinti; FDI = First dorsal interosseous.
* Concentric needle recording.

←——————————————————————————————————

Figure 3-6. Normal ulnar nerve motor response with stimulation at the wrist (A), below the elbow (B), above the elbow (C), at the axilla (D), and at Erb's point (E). Motor latencies and distances between stimulating and recording sites are indicated at each trace. Conduction velocities between consecutive stimulation sites are indicated between the respective traces.

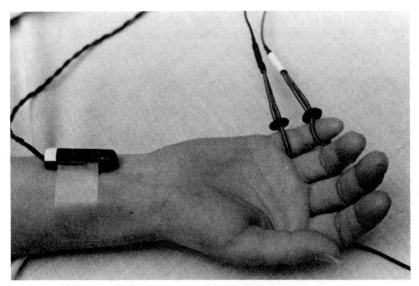

Figure 3-7. *Electrode placement for orthodromic recording of ulnar nerve sensory responses.*

Table 3-2. *Normal Values: Ulnar Orthodromic Sensory*

Parameter	Orthodromic digit V to wrist	Reference
Amplitude (μV) (peak to peak)	13.7 ± 6.4 (>5 μV)	[8]
Peak latency (msec) (distance 14.1 ± 0.6 cm)	2.8 ± 0.2 (<3.2)	[13]
Onset conduction velocity (m/sec)	60.9 ± 5.2 (>50.6)	[10]
Peak conduction velocity (m/sec)	47.5 ± 4.1 (>39.3)	[10]

Orthodromic Sensory

1. Stimulation (Fig. 3-7)
   a. Place the ring cathode near the fifth proximal interphalangeal joint.
   b. Place the ring anode around the fifth distal interphalangeal joint.
2. Ground is placed on the dorsum of the hand.
3. Recording electrode placement: G_1 end of the bar electrode is placed 10 to 14 cm proximal to the ring cathode over the ulnar nerve near the proximal wrist crease.

Normal values are listed in Table 3-2.

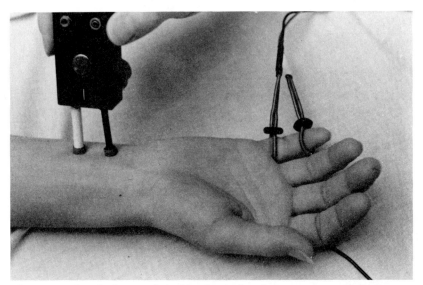

Figure 3-8. *Electrode placement for antidromic recording of ulnar nerve sensory responses.*

Table 3-3. *Normal Values: Ulnar Antidromic Sensory*

Parameter	Wrist to digit V	Below elbow to digit V	Above elbow to digit V	Reference
Amplitude (μV) (negative peak) (peak to peak)	35.0 ± 14.7 (>15 μV)	28.8 ± 12.2		[6] [7]
Peak latency (msec) (distance 14.1 ± 0.6 cm)	2.8 ± 0.2 (<3.2)			[13]
R-L latency difference (msec)	<0.4	<0.5	<0.8	[6]
Onset conduction velocity (m/sec)	54.8 ± 5.3 (>44.5)	64.7 ± 5.4 (>53.9)	66.7 ± 6.4 (>53.9)	[6]

Antidromic Sensory

1. Recording electrode placement (Fig. 3-8).
   a. G_1 ring electrode is placed near the fifth proximal interphalangeal joint.
   b. G_2 ring electrode is placed around the fifth distal interphalangeal joint.
2. Ground is placed on the dorsum of the hand.
3. Stimulate the ulnar nerve at the wrist near the proximal crease with the cathode 10 to 14 cm proximal to the G_1 ring electrode.

Normal values are listed in Table 3-3.

Table 3-4. *Normal Values: Ulnar Mixed Nerve Conduction*

Parameter	Stimulate at wrist record at elbow	Stimulate at elbow record at axilla	Stimulate at axilla record at Erb's point	Reference
Amplitude (μV) (peak to peak)	33.2 ± 14.8 >10 μV	34.8 ± 18.1 >10 μV	27.6 ± 14.2 >10 μV	[10]
Onset conduction velocity (m/sec)	68.4 ± 4.6 (>59.3)	73.1 ± 5.8 (>61.6)		[10]
Peak conduction velocity (m/sec)	55.4 ± 3.99 (>47.5)	57.2 ± 4.5 (>48.2)	64.1 ± 5.6 (>52.8)	[10]

Source: Values from Oh [10].

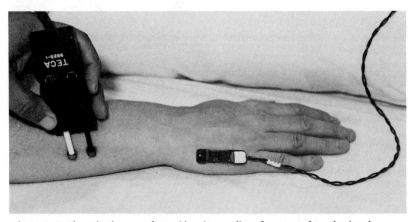

Figure 3-9. *Electrode placement for antidromic recording of responses from the dorsal cutaneous branch of the ulnar nerve. The ground electrode (not shown) is placed between the stimulating and recording electrodes.*

Mixed Nerve Conduction Studies

Mixed nerve conduction studies with stimulation at the wrist, elbow, and axilla (Table 3-4) are sometimes helpful in localizing proximal lesions. The electrodes are placed at the ulnar sulcus for recording mixed nerve potentials at the elbow.

Dorsal Cutaneous Branch (Antidromic Sensory)

The ulnar dorsal cutaneous nerve conduction study (Fig. 3-9, Table 3-5) is important because it is spared with ulnar nerve lesions at the

Table 3-5. *Normal Values: Ulnar Dorsal Cutaneous Branch*

Amplitude (peak to peak μV)	Peak latency (msec) (distance 8 cm)	Onset conduction velocity (m/sec)	Reference
20 ± 6 (>8)	2.0 ± 0.3 (<2.6)	60 ± 4.0 (>52)	[4]

Source: Values from Jabre [4].

wrist and therefore helps in localization. Isolated lesions of the nerve can occur as a result of tight wrist bands or handcuffs.

1. Recording electrode placement
   a. Place the G_1 active electrode at the apex of the V between the fourth and fifth metacarpal bones or on the fifth metacarpal bone (Fig. 3-9).
   b. Place the G_2 reference electrode distally at the base of the fifth digit.
2. Ground is placed between the stimulating and recording electrodes.
3. Stimulate the cathode 8 cm proximal to the G_1 electrode between the ulna and the flexor carpi ulnaris tendon (Fig. 3-9).

References

1. Bucthal, F., and Rosenfalck, A. Evoked action potentials and conduction velocity in human sensory nerves. *Brain Res.* 3:1, 1966.
2. Eisen, A. Early diagnosis of ulnar palsy: An electrophysiologic study. *Neurology (Minneap.)* 24:256, 1974.
3. Ginzberg, M., Lee, M., Ginzburg, J., et al. Median and ulnar nerve conduction determinations in the Erb's point-axilla segment in normal subjects. *J. Neurol. Neurosurg. Psychiatry* 41:444, 1978.
4. Jabre, J. F. Ulnar nerve lesions at wrist: New technique for recording from the sensory dorsal branch of the ulnar nerve. *Neurology (Minneap.)* 30:873, 1980.
5. Jebsen, R. H. Motor conduction velocities in the median and ulnar nerves. *Arch. Phys. Med. Rehabil.* 48:185, 1967.
6. Kimura, J. *Electrodiagnosis in Diseases of Nerve and Muscle: Principals and Practice.* Philadelphia: Davis, 1984.
7. Ma, D. M., and Liveson, J. A. *Nerve Conduction Handbook.* Philadelphia: Davis, 1983.
8. McLeod, J. G. Electrophysiological studies in the Guillain-Barré syndrome. *Ann. Neurol.* 9(Suppl.):20, 1981.
9. Miller, R. G. The cubital tunnel syndrome: diagnosis and precise localization. *Ann. Neurol.* 6:56, 1979.
10. Oh, S. J. *Clinical Electromyography: Nerve Conduction Studies.* Baltimore: University Park Press, 1984.
11. Olney, R. K., and Wilbourne, A. J. Ulnar nerve conduction study of the first dorsal interosseous muscle. *Arch. Phys. Med. Rehabil.* 66:16, 1985

12. Payan, J.   Electrophysiological localization of ulnar nerve lesions. *J. Neurol. Neurosurg. Psychiatry.* 32:208, 1969.
13. Rigshospitalet Laboratory of Clinical Neurophysiology. *Electromyography: Sensory and Motor Conduction. Findings in Normal Subjects.* Copenhagen: Rigshospitalet, 1975.

Median Nerve 4
Motor and Sensory Studies

Anatomy

The *median nerve* fibers ($C_{6,7,8}$ and T_1) pass through the upper, middle, and lower trunks and the lateral and medial cords of the brachial plexus (Fig. 4-1). The median nerve innervates the pronator teres before entering the forearm between the two heads of this muscle. It gives branches to the flexor carpi radialis, palmaris longus, and flexor digitorum sublimus and a purely motor branch, called the *anterior interos-*

Figure 4-1. *Origin and course of the median nerve.*

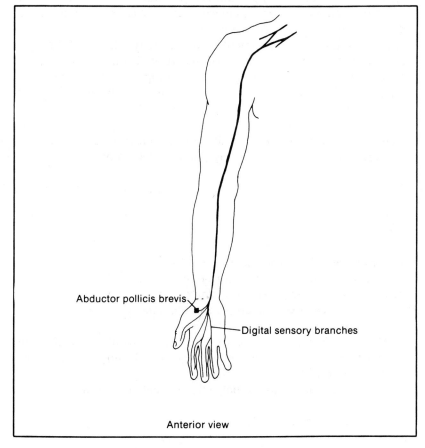

Abductor pollicis brevis

Digital sensory branches

Anterior view

seous nerve, which supplies the flexor pollicis longus, pronator quadratus, and the lateral half of the flexor digitorum profundus. The median nerve finally traverses the carpal tunnel under the flexor retinaculum from which it emerges to innervate the LOAF muscles of the hand (first and second *l*umbricals, *o*pponens pollicis, *a*bductor pollicis brevis, and *f*lexor pollicis brevis) as well as giving sensory branches to the volar surfaces of the lateral three and a half digits and the dorsal portion of their terminal phalanges.

Applications

Carpal tunnel syndrome is the most common entrapment neuropathy [1]. Proximal sites of entrapment are less frequent and include:

1. Ligament of Struther's syndrome [1,7]: compression of the median nerve under a fibrous band connecting an aberrant bony spur on the distal humerus to the medial epicondyle.
2. Pronator syndrome: entrapment between the two heads of the pronator teres by a tendinous band or hypertrophied muscle [1].
3. Anterior interosseous nerve syndrome: entrapment at the tendinous origin of muscles or an aberrant vessel 5 to 8 cm below the elbow [1].

Thenar wasting can be seen in the thoracic outlet syndrome due to involvement of fibers that ultimately join the median nerve.

Procedure
Motor

1. Recording electrode placement (Fig. 4.2)
   a. G_1 is placed over the abductor pollicis brevis.
   b. G_2 is placed over proximal phalanx of the thumb.
2. Ground is placed over the dorsum of the hand.
3. Stimulation
   a. Midwrist: Palmar aspect, between the tendons of the flexor carpi radialis (laterally) and palmaris longus (medially), with the cathode 6.5 cm proximal to G_1 (Fig. 4-2).
   b. Elbow: just medial to the palpable brachial artery (Fig. 4-3).
   c. Axilla (see Fig. 2-8).
   d. Erb's point (see Fig. 2-9).

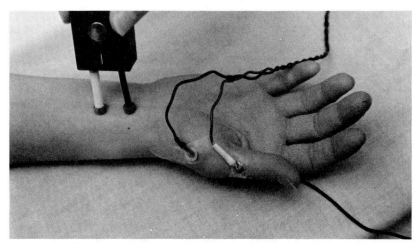

Figure 4-2. *Electrode placement for recording from the abductor pollicis brevis and stimulation of the median nerve at the wrist.*

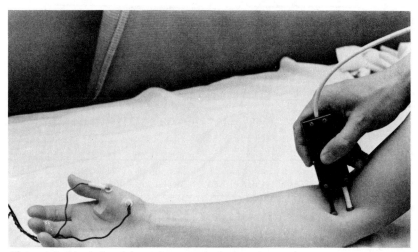

Figure 4-3. *Stimulation of the median nerve in the antecubital fossa.*

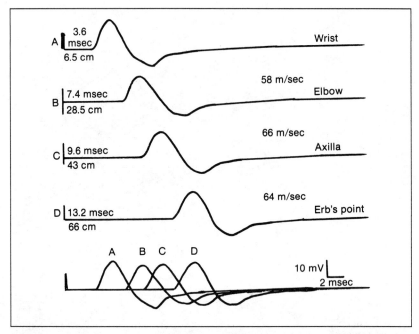

Figure 4-4. *Normal median motor responses with stimulation at the wrist* (A), *elbow* (B), *axilla* (C), *and Erb's point* (D). *The distances are from the cathode to the active recording electrode. The indicated latencies are from each stimulation site and the conduction velocities are between consecutive stimulation sites.*

Table 4-1. *Normal Values: Median Motor*

Segment	Distal latency or NCV	Amplitude peak to peak (mV)	Reference
Wrist to APB		15.8 ± 5.9 (>5 mV)	[9] [4,9,14,15]
Wrist to APB (distance 6.5 cm)	3.2 ± 0.3 (2.5–3.8) msec		[16]
R-L latency difference (wrist) (msec)	(<0.7)		[6]
Elbow to wrist	58.5 ± 4.54 (49.7–69.1) msec		[9,10]
Axilla to elbow	65.3 ± 3.47 (57.3–71.9) m/sec		[9]
Erb's point to axilla	65.1 ± 6.1 (57.1–76.2) m/sec	[3]	
Erb's point to elbow	62.8 ± 6.0 (53–77) msec		[5]

APB = abductor pollicis brevis.

Figure 4-4 illustrates normal motor responses from stimulation at these sites and Table 4-1 lists the normal values.

THE MARTIN-GRUBER ANASTOMOSIS. In about 15 to 30 percent of the population, axons to the ulnar-innervated intrinsic hand muscles cross in the forearm from the median nerve, or one of its branches, to the ulnar nerve. This anomalous median-to-ulnar anastomosis is inherited as an autosomal dominant trait and is bilateral in two-thirds of patients. It is recognized electrophysiologically by a higher amplitude and an initial positivity (downward deflection) of the median motor response with stimulation at the elbow when compared to the motor response with wrist stimulation. The ulnar motor response is smaller at the elbow than at the wrist.

Orthodromic Sensory

1. Stimulation (Fig. 4-5)
   a. Ring cathode is placed near the second proximal interphalangeal joint.
   b. Ring anode is placed around the second distal interphalangeal joint.
2. Ground is placed on the dorsum of the hand.
3. Recording electrode placement: G_1 end of the bar electrode is placed

Figure 4-5. *Electrode placement for orthodromic recording of median nerve sensory responses.*

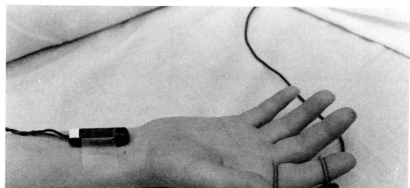

Table 4-2. *Normal Values: Median Orthodromic Sensory*

Parameter	Digit II to wrist	Palm to wrist	Reference
Amplitude (μV) peak to peak	30.9 ± 12.1 (>10 μV)	71.4 ± 37.9 (>10 μV)	[15]
Median/ulnar amplitude ratio	1.5 ± 0.36 (>1.1)		[8,11]
Peak latency (msec) (distance 14 cm)	3.0 ± 0.25 (<3.5)	(<2.2)	[13,17]
Onset conduction velocity (m/sec)	60.9 ± 5.07 (>50)	58.6 ± 6.0 (>46.6)	[10,15]
Peak conduction velocity (m/sec)	49.5 ± 4.14 (>41.3)	41.9 ± 3.9 (>34.1)	[15]

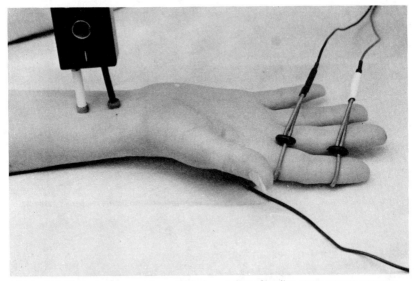

Figure 4-6. *Electrode placement for antidromic recording of median nerve sensory responses.*

over the median nerve on the anterior aspect of the wrist 14 cm proximal to the ring cathode.

Normal values are listed in Table 4-2.

Antidromic Sensory

1. Recording electrode placement (Fig. 4-6)
    a. G₁ ring is placed near the second proximal interphalangeal joint.
    b. G₂ ring is placed around the second distal interphalangeal joint.
2. Ground is placed on the dorsum of the hand.

Table 4-3. *Normal Values: Median Antidromic Sensory*

Parameter	Elbow to digit II	Wrist to digit II	Palm to digit II	Reference
Amplitude (μV) peak to peak	>7	>16	>32	[9,14]
Peak latency (msec) Wrist to digit II (14 cm) Palm to digit II (7 cm)		3.2 ± 0.25 (<3.7)	1.8 ± 0.19 (<2.2)	[2,13]
R-L latency difference (wrist) (msec)		(<0.5)		[6]
Onset conduction velocity (m/sec)	61.8 ± 4.2 (>53)	57.4 ± 3.8 (>49.8)	58.8 ± 5.8 (>47)	[6,13]
Peak conduction velocity (m/sec)		44.0 ± 4.0 (36–56)		[12]

Table 4-4. *Normal Values: Median Mixed Nerve Conduction*

Parameter	Stimulate at wrist record at elbow	Stimulate at elbow record at axilla	Reference
Amplitude (μV) peak to peak	32.1 ± 16.3 (>10)	44.5 ± 19 (>10)	[15]
Onset conduction velocity (m/sec)	64.5 ± 4.3 (>55.9)	74.8 ± 4.8 (>65.3)	[15]
Peak conduction velocity (m/sec)	56.0 ± 3.3 (>49.4)	63.5 ± 4.8 (>54.0)	[15]

Source: Values from Oh [15].

3. Stimulate over the median nerve at the midwrist anteriorly, near the proximal crease, with the cathode 12 to 14 cm proximal to the G_1 ring electrode.

Normal values are listed in Table 4-3.

Mixed Nerve Conduction Studies
Mixed nerve conduction studies (Table 4-4) are useful in localizing proximal lesions because sensory responses are very small at proximal recording sites.

References

1. Dawson, D. M., Hallet, M., and Millender, L. H.   Entrapment Neuropathies. Boston: Little, Brown, 1983.
2. Felsenthal, G., and Spindler, H.   Palmar conduction time of median and ulnar nerves of normal subjects and patients with carpal tunnel syndrome. *Am. J. Phys. Med.* 58:131, 1979.
3. Ginzburg, M., Lee, M., Ginzburg, J., et al.   Median and ulnar nerve conduction determinations in the Erb's point-axilla segment in normal subjects. *J. Neurol. Neurosurg. Psychiatry* 41:444, 1978.
4. Hodes, R., Larrabee, M. G., and German, W.   The human electromyogram in response to nerve stimulation and conduction velocity of motor axons. *Arch. Neurol. Psychiatry* 60:340, 1948.
5. Jebsen, R. H.   Motor conduction velocities in the median and ulnar nerves. *Arch. Phys. Med. Rehabil.* 48:185, 1967.
6. Kimura, J.   *Electrodiagnosis in Diseases of Nerve and Muscle: Principals and Practice.* Philadelphia: Davis, 1984.
7. Kopell, P., and Thompson, W. A. L.   *Peripheral Entrapment Neuropathies.* Baltimore: Williams & Wilkins, 1963.
8. Loong, S. C., and Seah, C. S.   Comparison of median and ulnar sensory action potentials in the diagnosis of the carpal tunnel syndrome. *J. Neurol. Neurosurg. Psychiatry* 34:750, 1971.
9. Ma, D. M., and Liveson, J. A.   *Nerve Conduction Handbook.* Philadelphia: Davis, 1983.
10. McLeod, J. G., Morgan, J. A., and Reye, C.   Electrophysiologic studies in familial spastic paraplegia. *J. Neurol. Neurosurg. Psychiatry* 40:611, 1977.
11. Martinez, A. C., et al.   Electrophysiological aspects of sensory conduction velocity in healthy adults. Part 2. Ratio between the amplitude of sensory evoked potentials at the wrist on stimulating different fingers in both hands. *J. Neurol. Neurosurg. Psychiatry* 41:1097, 1978.
12. Mavor, H., and Shiozawa, R.   Antidromic digital and palmar nerve action potentials. *Electroencephalogr. Clin. Neurophysiol.* 30:210, 1971.
13. Melvin, J. L., Harris, D. H., and Johnson, E. W.   Sensory and motor conduction velocities in the ulnar and median nerves. *Arch. Phys. Med. Rehabil.* 47:511, 1966.
14. Melvin, J. L., Schuchmann, J. A., and Lanese, R. R.   Diagnostic specificity of motor and sensory nerve conduction variables in the carpal tunnel syndrome. *Arch. Phys. Med. Rehabil.* 54:69, 1973.
15. Oh, S. J.   *Clinical Electromyography: Nerve Conduction Studies.* Baltimore: University Park Press, 1984.
16. Rigshospitalet Laboratory of Clinical Neurophysiology. *Electromyography: Sensory and Motor Conduction. Findings in Normal Subjects.* Copenhagen: Rigshospitalet, 1975.
17. Stevens, J. C.   AAEE Minimonograph #26: The electrodiagnosis of carpal tunnel syndrome. *Muscle Nerve* 10:99, 1987.

Radial Nerve 5
Motor and Sensory Studies

Anatomy

The *radial nerve* receives contributions mainly from $C_{5,6,7,8}$ which pass through the upper, middle, and lower trunks and posterior cord of the brachial plexus. The radial nerve is the largest terminal branch of the brachial plexus and supplies the extensor muscles of the arm and forearm (Fig. 5-1) as well as the skin covering them. The radial nerve gives branches to the triceps and anconeus muscles before winding around

Figure 5-1. *Origin and course of the radial nerve.*

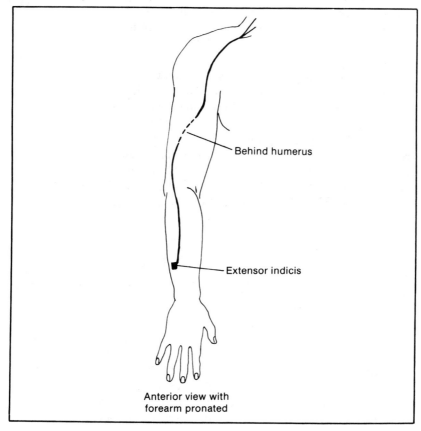

Behind humerus

Extensor indicis

Anterior view with
forearm pronated

the humerus in the *spiral groove*. Motor fibers to the brachioradialis, extensor carpi radialis longus and brevis, and supinator muscles arise prior to the radial nerve's entrance into the posterior compartment of the forearm through the fibrous arch of the supinator muscle (*arcade of Frohse*). The radial nerve then continues as the *posterior interosseous nerve*, which innervates the remaining wrist and finger extensors. It becomes superficial about 8 cm proximal to the ulnar styloid on the ulnar aspect of the forearm before finally terminating in the extensor indicis proprius. The *superficial radial nerve* (C_6 or C_7 roots) separates from the main trunk slightly above the lateral aspect of the elbow and descends to the distal forearm where it becomes superficial and supplies the radial aspect of the hand and the proximal dorsum of the first three and a half digits (Fig. 5-4).

Applications

The most common site for radial nerve lesions is at the spiral groove where it lies against the bone. Radial neuropathy at this site is most often due to external compression against the humeral shaft (e.g., "Saturday night" palsy) but may also be associated with fractures of the humerus.

Posterior interosseous syndrome is an infrequent entrapment at the fibrous arch of origin of the supinator muscle resulting in weakness of the finger extensor muscles and the extensor carpi ulnaris. A syndrome similar to lateral epicondylitis ("resistant tennis elbow") may on occasion be due to posterior interosseus nerve entrapment, resulting from repeated forced supination of the arm. Isolated lesions of the superficial radial nerve are seen with compression from tight wrist bands ("handcuff neuropathy"). Finally, radial sensory nerve conduction studies are important in trying to differentiate a C_6 and C_7 root lesion from a plexus lesion.

Procedure
Motor

1. Recording electrode placement
    a. A concentric needle electrode is placed in the extensor indicis proprius muscle which can be palpated along the dorsal ulnar aspect of the forearm 4 to 6 cm proximal to the ulnar styloid when the patient extends the index finger. Needle recordings of more proximal muscles such as the extensor digitorum communis or the brachioradialis are also commonly used to compute the conduction

velocity in the spiral groove (axilla–to–above elbow segment), which is the most frequent site of injury.

b. Surface electrode recordings may be tried with the G_1 electrode over the extensor indicis proprius and the G_2 electrode over the ulnar styloid (Fig. 5-2).

2. Ground is placed close to the recording electrode (Figs. 5-2, 5-3).

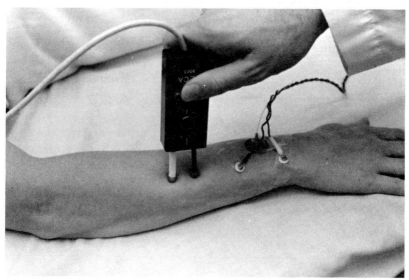

Figure 5-2. *Electrode placement for recording from the extensor indicis proprius and distal stimulation of the radial nerve (motor).*

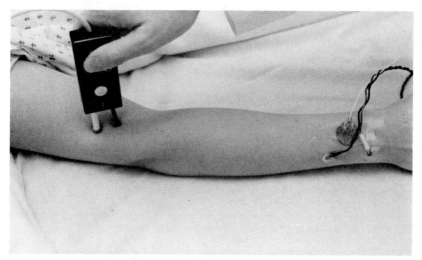

Figure 5-3. *Proximal stimulation of the radial nerve (motor) in the antecubital fossa.*

3. Stimulation
   a. Forearm: approximately 8 cm proximal to the ulnar styloid just radial to the extensor carpi ulnaris muscle (Fig. 5-2).
   b. Elbow: in the groove between the brachioradialis muscle and the biceps tendon, about 6 cm proximal to the lateral epicondyle of the humerus (Fig. 5-3).
   c. Axilla: just posterior to the palpable axillary artery in the groove between the corachobrachialis anteriorly and triceps posteriorly (see Fig. 2-8).
   d. Erb's point (see Fig. 2-9).
4. Distance measurements for Erb's-axilla and axilla-elbow segments are done with an obstetric caliper. Anterior surface tape measurement across the biceps for the axilla-elbow segment may be equally accurate [3].

Normal values are listed in Table 5-1.

The conduction velocity between axilla and elbow is the same whether measured in fibers to the brachioradialis, extensor digitorum communis or the extensor indicis proprius [8].

Table 5-1. *Normal Values: Radial Motor*

Segment	Distal latency (msec) or NCV (m/sec)	Amplitude (mV) (peak to peak)	Reference
Forearm to EIP (6.2 ± 0.9 cm)	2.4 ± 0.5 (<2.9)	14 ± 8.8	[8][a]
Elbow to EDC (distance 11 cm)	3.1 (2.5–3.6)	(7–31)	[6][a]
Elbow to brachioradialis (distance 9 cm)	2.6 (2.0–3.1)	(7–30)	[6][a]
Axilla to triceps (distance 11 cm)	2.9 (1.8–3.2)	(11–35)	[6][a]
Erb's point to triceps (distance 25–28 cm)	4.5 ± 0.45 (<5.3)		[1][a]
Elbow to forearm	62 ± 5.1 (>51.8)	13 ± 8.2	[8][a]
Axilla to elbow	69 ± 5.6 (>57.8)	11 ± 7.0	[8][a]
Erb's point to elbow	72 ± 6.3 (56–93)	10.5 (8–14)	[2][b]

EIP = extensor indicis proprius; EDC = extensor digitorum communis.
[a] Concentric needle recording electrode.
[b] Surface recording electrode.

Antidromic Sensory

1. Recording electrode placement
    a. Place the G_1 electrode over the palpable superficial radial nerve as it crosses the tendon of the extensor pollicis longus on the ulnar side of the anatomic snuffbox (Figs. 5-4, 5-5).
    b. Place the G_2 electrode 3 cm distal to G_1.
2. Ground is placed close to the recording electrodes (Fig. 5-5).

Figure 5-4. *Terminal course of the superficial radial nerve.*

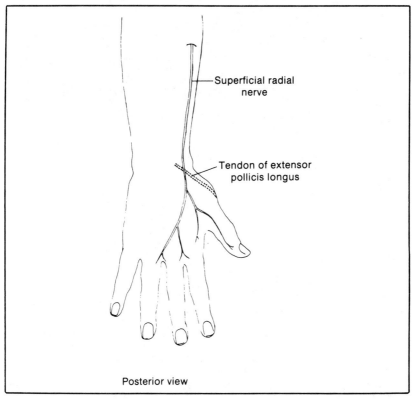

Superficial radial nerve

Tendon of extensor pollicis longus

Posterior view

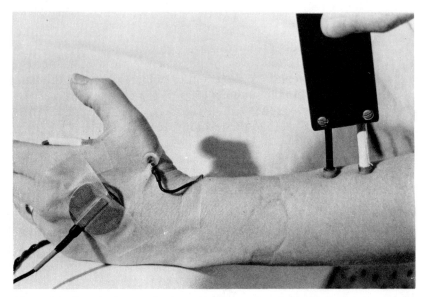

Figure 5-5. *Electrode placement for the antidromic recording of superficial radial nerve sensory responses.*

Table 5-2. *Normal Values: Radial Antidromic Sensory*

Segment	Forearm to wrist	Reference
Amplitude (peak to peak) (μV)	21.4 ± 4.8 (15–35)	[7]
Onset latency (msec) (distance 10 cm)	1.8 ± 0.15 (<2.1)	[4]
Peak latency (msec) (distance 10 cm)	2.3 ± 0.2 (<2.7)	[4]
Peak latency (msec) (distance 14 cm)	2.9 ± 0.2 (<3.3)	[4]
Onset conduction velocity (m/sec)	58.1 ± 4.7 (50–68)	[7]
Peak conduction velocity (m/sec)	50.9 ± 3.28 (>44.3)	[5]

3. Stimulate with the cathode 10 to 14 cm proximal to the G_1 electrode over the radial aspect of the forearm (Fig. 5-5).

Normal values are listed in Table 5-2.

References

1. Gassel, M. M., and Diamantopoulos, E.   Pattern of conduction times in the distribution of the radial nerve: A clinical and electrophysiological study. *Neurology (Minneap.)* 14:222, 1964.
2. Jebsen, R. H.   Motor conduction velocity in proximal and distal segments of the radial nerve. *Arch. Phys. Med. Rehabil.* 47:597, 1966.
3. Kalyantri, A., et al.   Axilla-to-elbow radial nerve conduction. *Muscle Nerve* 11:133, 1988.
4. Mackenzie, K., and DeLisa, J. A.   Distal sensory latency measurement of the superficial radial nerve in normal adult subjects. *Arch. Phys. Med. Rehabil.* 62:31, 1981.
5. Oh, S. J.   *Clinical Electromyography: Nerve Conduction Studies.* Baltimore: University Park Press, 1984.
6. Rigshospitalet Laboratory of Clinical Neurophysiology. *Electromyography: Sensory and Motor Conduction. Findings in Normal Subjects.* Copenhagen: Rigshospitalet, 1975.
7. Shahani, B., Goodgold, J., and Spielholz, N. I.   Sensory nerve action potential in the radial nerve. *Arch. Phys. Med. Rehabil.* 48:602, 1967.
8. Trojaburg, W., and Sindrup, G. H.   Motor and sensory conduction in different segments of the radial nerve in normal subjects. *J. Neurol. Neurosurg. Psychiatry* 32:354, 1969.

Musculocutaneous Nerve **6**
Sensory Studies

Anatomy

The *musculocutaneous nerve* receives fibers from $C_{5,6,7}$ that pass through the upper and middle trunks and the lateral cord of the brachial plexus (see Fig. 2-1). The musculocutaneous nerve provides motor innervation to the biceps, brachialis, and corachobrachialis (BBC) and supplies the

Figure 6-1. *Superficial course of the lateral antebrachial cutaneous branch of the musculocutaneous nerve in the forearm.*

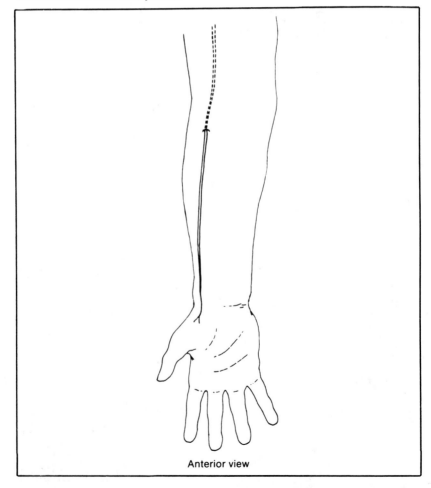

Anterior view

skin over the radial aspect of the forearm as the *lateral antebrachial cutaneous nerve* (Fig. 6-1). The sensory fibers originate mainly from the C_6 root and travel via the upper trunk and lateral cord of the brachial plexus.

Applications

Study results are useful in analyzing isolated lesions of the musculocutaneous nerve and aid in distinguishing C_6 radiculopathies from lesions of the upper trunk of the brachial plexus. Sensory responses may be obtainable in peripheral polyneuropathies after it is no longer possible to obtain ulnar and median sensory responses [1].

Procedure
Antidromic Sensory

1. Recording electrode placement
    a. G_1 recording electrode is placed 12 cm distal to the cathode along a line connecting the stimulation point to the radial styloid (Fig. 6-2).
    b. G_2 reference electrode is placed 3 cm distal to G_1 (Fig. 6-2).
2. Ground is placed close to the recording electrodes (Fig. 6-2).

Figure 6-2. *Electrode placement for antidromic recording of the lateral antebrachial cutaneous branch of the musculocutaneous nerve.*

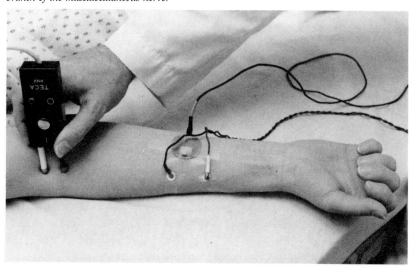

Table 6-1. *Normal Values: Lateral Antebrachial Antidromic Sensory*

Parameter	Elbow to wrist	Reference
Amplitude (peak to peak) (μV)	24.0 ± 7.2 (12–50)	[2]
Onset latency (msec) (distance 12 cm)	1.8 ± 0.1 (1.6–2.1)	[2]
Peak latency (msec) (distance 12 cm)	2.3 ± 0.1 (2.2–2.6)	[2]
Onset (maximum) conduction velocity (m/sec)	65.0 ± 3.6 (57–75)	[2]

Source: Values from Spindler [2].

3. Stimulation: Place the cathode of the stimulating electrode in the elbow crease immediately lateral to the biceps tendon (Fig. 6-2).

Normal values are listed in Table 6-1.

References
1. Lambert, E. H., and Daube, J. R. (Chairmen). *Special Course #16: Clinical Electromyography*. American Academy of Neurology Meeting, Chicago, Ill. April 23–28, 1979.
2. Spindler, H. A., and Felsenthal, G. Sensory conduction in the musculocutaneous nerve. *Arch. Phys. Med. Rehabil.* 59:20, 1978.

Sciatic Nerve, Lumbosacral 7
Roots, and Plexus
Motor Studies

Anatomy

The *spinal nerves* in the lumbosacral region exit from the intervertebral foramina inferior to the vertebra of the same number and immediately split into the dorsal and ventral rami (see Fig. 18-20). The dorsal rami supply the paraspinal muscles and skin of the dorsal part of the trunk. The ventral rami form the lumbosacral plexus (Fig. 7-1).

The *sciatic nerve* is the largest nerve in the body and receives contributions from the $L_{4,5}$ and $S_{1,2,3}$ spinal nerves. It exits the pelvis through the greater sciatic notch beneath the tendinous origin of the piriformis muscle. At the gluteal fold, the sciatic nerve is accessible to transcutaneous stimulation (Fig. 7-2).

The sciatic nerve is actually two nerves within a common sheath: the common peroneal (laterally placed) and the tibial (medially placed) nerves, which separate at a variable distance above the popliteal fossa. The sciatic nerve conveys cutaneous sensation from the posterolateral leg and the foot and provides motor innervation to all the muscles of the leg and foot through the common peroneal and tibial branches. Nerves to the semitendinosus, semimembranosus, biceps femoris (long head), and adductor magnus are direct branches of the tibial division of the sciatic trunk, whereas the peroneal division in the thigh only supplies the short head of the biceps.

Applications

Sciatic nerve injury is often secondary to pelvic or femoral fractures, hip dislocations, surgery, or direct injection into the nerve. Compression of the sciatic nerve within the pelvis occurs with retroperitoneal bleeding or tumors. Entrapment of the sciatic nerve has been observed against the tendinous origin of the piriformis muscle at the sciatic notch (piriformis syndrome) [1]. Ischemic mononeuropathy is seen in diabetics and in patients with collagen vascular diseases.

Sciatic nerve lesions need to be differentiated from lesions of the cauda equina, lumbosacral plexus, common peroneal, and tibial nerves. In combination with peroneal and tibial nerve studies, conduction studies in the sciatic nerve and lumbosacral plexus may help in localization.

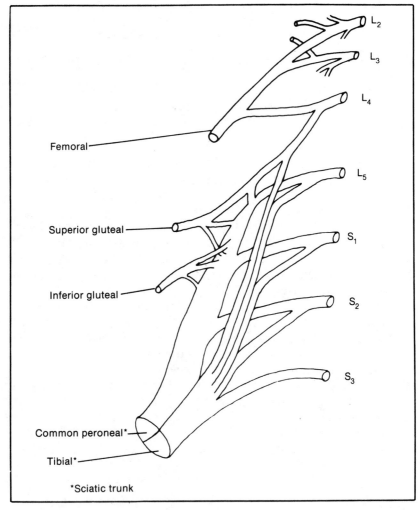

Figure 7-1. *Simplified plan of the lumbosacral plexus emphasizing commonly studied nerves.*

Procedure
Sciatic Nerve

1. Recording electrode placement
   a. G_1 is placed over the abductor digiti quini (Fig. 7-3) or abductor hallucis (see Fig. 10-2).
   b. G_2 over the corresponding toe. Other sciatic nerve–innervated muscles like the extensor digitorum brevis, tibialis anterior, or gastrocnemius can also be used. Needle electrode recordings are nec-

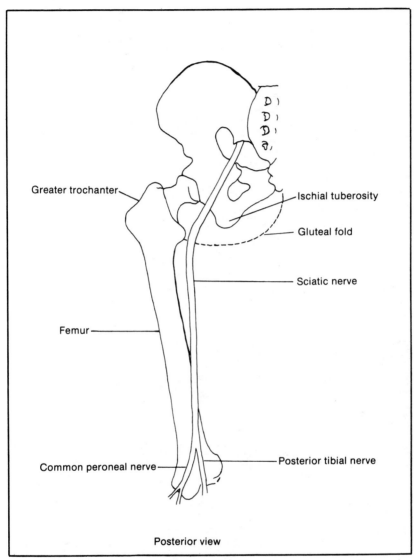

Figure 7-2. *Landmarks for locating the superficial portion of the sciatic nerve trunk.*

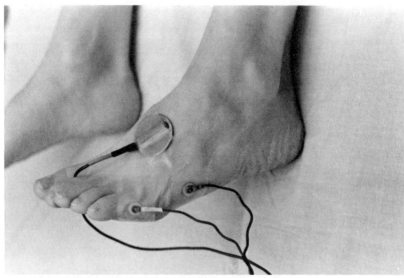

Figure 7-3. *Recording electrode placement for recording from the abductor digiti quinti (lateral plantar branch of the posterior tibial nerve) in sciatic nerve conduction studies.*

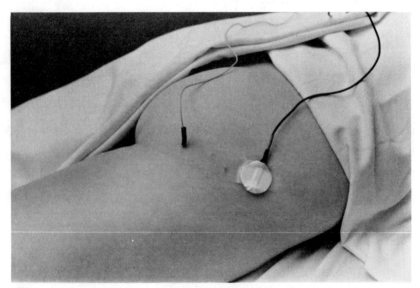

Figure 7-4. *Stimulation of the sciatic nerve at the gluteal fold.*

essary for proximal muscles to avoid picking up volume-conducted potential from neighboring muscles.
2. Ground is placed on the dorsum of the foot.
3. Stimulation
    a. *Transcutaneous-sciatic*: The cathode is a 50 to 75-mm monopolar EMG needle inserted in the gluteal skin fold equidistant from the ischial tuberosity and the greater trochanter of the femur. The disc anode is placed on the nearby skin (see Fig. 7-4).
    b. *Percutaneous (tibial)*: The cathode is placed in the middle of the popliteal fossa (Fig. 7-5).

The amplitude of responses from distal stimulation is generally above 5 mV. The conduction velocity is generally higher when proximal leg muscles are used for recording (Table 7-1).

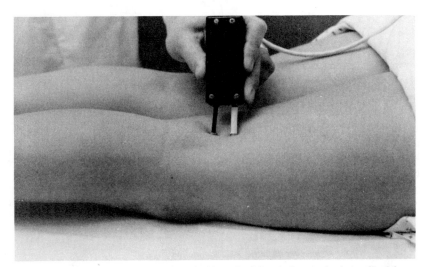

Figure 7-5. *Stimulation of the posterior tibial branch of the sciatic nerve in the popliteal fossa.*

Table 7-1. *Normal Values: Sciatic Nerve*

Segment	NCV (m/sec)	Reference
Gluteal fold to popliteal fossa (recording at ADQ)	51.3 ± 4.4 (45.3–61.1)	[6]
Gluteal fold to popliteal fossa (recording at gastrocnemius)	53.8 ± 3.3 (49.2–60.7)	[6]
Gluteal fold to ankle	48.0 ± 3.5 (>41)	[2]

ADQ = abductor digiti quinti.

Lumbosacral Roots

For transcutaneous stimulation of the lumbosacral roots (Fig. 7-6), insert the cathode (75-mm monopolar EMG needle) perpendicularly in the paraspinal region just medial and slightly caudal to the posterior iliac spine to stimulate the S_1 root; at the level of the iliac crest for the L_4 root; and in between these two points for the L_5 root. Appropriate root-innervated muscles are chosen for recording (e.g., abductor hallucis for the S_1 root, tibialis anterior for the L_5 root, and vastus medialis for the

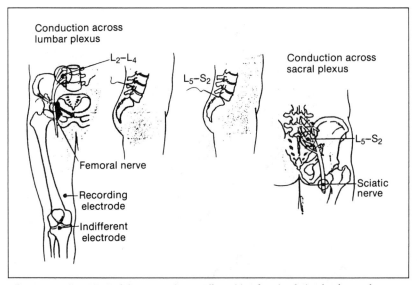

Figure 7-6. *Illustration of the appropriate needle position for stimulating lumbosacral roots. (From I. C. MacLean. Nerve root stimulation to evaluate conduction across the brachial and lumbosacral plexus.* Third Annual Continuing Education Course. *American Association of Electromyography and Electrodiagnosis, Philadelphia, PA, 1980. Used by permission.)*

Table 7-2. *Normal Values: Lumbosacral Root Stimulation*

Segment	Latency (m/sec)	Reference
S_1 to soleus	15.4 ± 1.3	[3]
Ratio S_1/H-reflex latency	47.1 ± 2.3%	[3]
S_1 to soleus R-L latency difference	<1 msec	[4]
S_1 tp gluteal fold[a]	3.9 ± 0.7 (2.5–4.9)	[5]
L_4 to inguinal region[b]	3.4 ± 0.6 (2.0–4.4)	[5]

[a] Subtraction of S_1 from sciatic nerve latency with recording from abductor hallucis.
[b] Subtraction of S_1 from femoral nerve latency (see Chapter 12) with recording from vastus medialis.

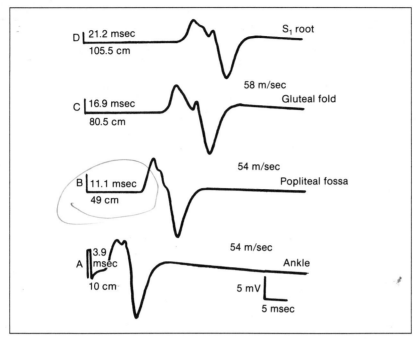

Figure 7-7. *Normal CMAP from the abductor hallucis with stimulation of the tibial nerve at the ankle (A) and popliteal fossa (B); sciatic nerve at the gluteal fold (C); and S₁ root in the paraspinal region (D). Distances are between the cathode and active recording electrode. The latency from each stimulation site is indicated above the respective trace. The conduction velocities are between consecutive stimulation sites.*

L_4 root). Conduction time across the plexus can be calculated by subtracting the proximal latency obtained by root stimulation from a distal latency obtained by stimulating the sciatic or femoral nerve distal to the plexus (Table 7-2).

A typical normal motor response obtained from the S_1 root, sciatic nerve, and tibial nerve stimulation is shown in Figure 7-7.

References

1. Dawson, D. M., Hallet, M., and Millender, L. H. *Entrapment Neuropathies.* Boston: Little, Brown, 1983.
2. Gassel, M. M., and Trojaborg, W. Clinical and electrophysiological study of the pattern of conduction times in the distribution of the sciatic nerve. *J. Neurol. Neurosurg. Psychiatry* 27:351, 1964.
3. Johnson, E. W. Spinal Nerve Stimulation. Thirty-Third Annual Meeting, Didactic Program, American Association of Electromyography and Electrodiagnosis, Boston, MA., September 25, 1986.
4. Johnson, E. W., Pease, W., Gatens, P., et al. Combination of H-reflex and

S$_1$ spinal nerve stimulation in S$_1$ radiculopathy. *Arch. Phys. Med. Rehabil.* 66:546, 1985.
5. MacLean, I. C. Nerve root stimulation to evaluate conduction across the brachial and lumbosacral plexuses. *Third Annual Continuing Education Course.* American Association of Electromyography and Electrodiagnosis, Philadelphia, PA. September 25, 1980.
6. Yap, C. P., and Hirota, T. Sciatic nerve motor conduction velocity study. *J. Neurol. Neurosurg. Psychiatry* 30:233, 1967.

Peroneal Nerve 8
Motor Studies

Anatomy

The *common peroneal nerve* ($L_{4,5}$,$S_{1,2}$) runs laterally in the popliteal fossa after its origin from the sciatic nerve, winding around the neck of the fibula and dividing into the superficial and deep peroneal nerves. The *deep peroneal nerve* descends deep in the anterior compartment of the leg and provides motor innervation to the dorsiflexors of the foot and toes. It becomes superficial just above the ankle before passing under the extensor retinaculum and dividing into terminal, medial, and lateral branches. The lateral (motor) branch innervates the extensor digitorum brevis and the medial (sensory) branch terminates in the first dorsal web space. The *superficial peroneal division* provides motor innervation to the peroneus longus and peroneus brevis muscles and sensory innervation to the lower lateral leg and dorsum of the foot (Fig. 8-1).

Applications

The common peroneal nerve is vulnerable to compression where it becomes superficial over the lateral aspect of the neck of the fibula. Injury to the peroneal nerve at this level causes a foot drop with impaired dorsiflexion and eversion of the foot. Slowing of the conduction velocity by greater than 10 m/sec across the fibular head is useful for localization.

Less commonly, a proximal sciatic lesion can selectively affect the peroneal fibers. These patients have involvement of the biceps femoris (short head) in addition to the peroneal nerve innervated muscles.

An L_5 radiculopathy can also cause weakness and sensory disturbance in the peroneal nerve distribution. These patients have additional involvement of the foot invertors, and the peroneal sensory response is preserved in spite of sensory loss because the lesion here is preganglionic. The peroneal nerve is also involved early in generalized polyneuropathies.

Procedure

1. Recording electrode placement (Fig. 8-2)
   a. G_1 recording electrode is placed over the extensor digitorum brevis muscle
   b. G_2 recording electrode is placed over the fifth toe

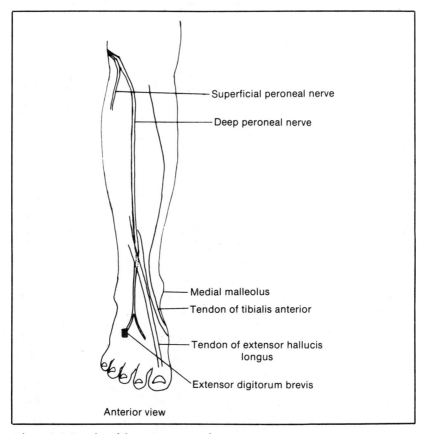

Superficial peroneal nerve

Deep peroneal nerve

Medial malleolus

Tendon of tibialis anterior

Tendon of extensor hallucis longus

Extensor digitorum brevis

Anterior view

Figure 8-1. Branches of the common peroneal nerve.

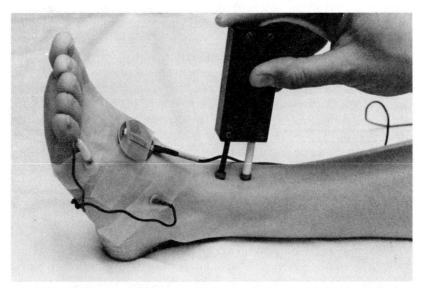

Figure 8-2. Electrode placement for recording from the extensor digitorum brevis and distal stimulation of the deep peroneal nerve.

2. Ground is placed close to the recording electrodes
3. Stimulation
   a. Dorsal aspect of distal lower leg between the tendons of the tibialis anterior (medially) and the extensor hallucis (laterally), 9 cm proximal to the active recording electrode (Fig. 8-2)
   b. 3 to 4 cm distal to the proximal tip of the fibular head (Fig. 8-3)
   c. Lateral popliteal fossa, medial to the biceps femoris tendon (Fig. 8-4)

Normal values are listed in Table 8-1.

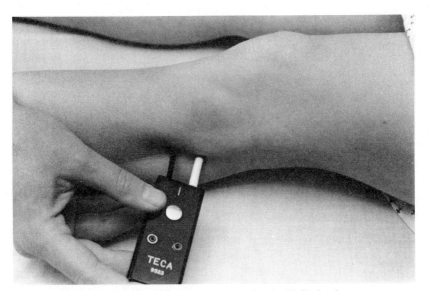

Figure 8-3. Stimulation of the peroneal nerve just distal to the fibular head.

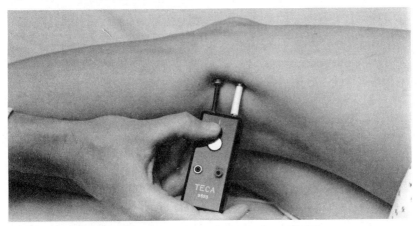

Figure 8-4. Stimulation of the common peroneal nerve in the popliteal fossa.

Table 8-1. *Normal Values: Peroneal Motor*

Segment	Latency (msec) or NCV (m/sec)	Amplitude peak to peak (mV)	Reference
Ankle to EDB		10.1 ± 4.8 (>4)	[2]
Ankle to EDB (distance 9 cm)	4.1 ± 0.4 (3.4–5.0)		[3]
Ankle to EDB R-L latency difference	<1.84		[1]
Below fibula head* to tibialis anterior or peroneus longus (distance 10 cm)	3.0 ± 0.35 (2.3–3.7)	15.0 (6–34)	[3]
Above fibula head to ankle	51.0 ± 3.5 (44–57)		[3]
Below fibula head to ankle	50.0 ± 3.5 (43–57)		[3]
Across fibula head (11 cm) (recording at EDB)	49.0 ± 4.0 (41–58)		[3]
Across fibula head (11 cm) (recording at tibialis anterior or peroneus longus)	58.0 (50–69)		[3]

EDB = extensor digitorum brevis.
* Concentric needle recording.

Figure 8-5. *Normal motor responses from the extensor digitorum brevis with stimulation of the peroneal nerve at the ankle (A), fibular head (B), and popliteal fossa (C). The latency indicated at each trace is from the respective stimulation site. The conduction velocities are between consecutive stimulation sites.*

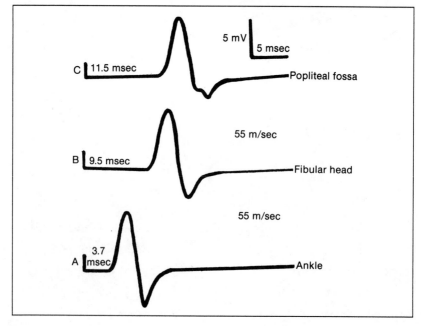

Figure 8-5 shows normal motor responses with stimulation at all three sites.

In about 20 percent of the population the lateral portion of the extensor digitorum brevis is supplied by an *accessory deep peroneal nerve* which may be stimulated behind the lateral malleolus. These patients are recognized by having a higher amplitude response on proximal stimulation.

References

1. Kimura, J.   *Electrodiagnosis in Diseases of Nerve and Muscle: Principles and Practice*. Philadelphia: Davis, 1984.
2. Oh, S. J.   *Clinical Electromyography: Nerve Conduction Studies*. Baltimore: University Park Press, 1984.
3. Rigshospitalet Laboratory of Clinical Neurophysiology. *Electromyography: Sensory and Motor Conduction. Findings in Normal Subjects*. Copenhagen: Rigshospitalet, 1975.

Superficial Peroneal Nerve 9
Sensory Studies

Anatomy

The *superficial peroneal nerve* receives its sensory fibers mainly from the L₅ root. It separates from the common peroneal nerve just distal to the fibular head, passes distally, pierces the deep fascia in the lower third of the leg, and divides into the *medial* and *intermediate dorsal cutaneous nerves* (Fig. 9-1). The superficial peroneal nerve supplies sensation to the lower lateral leg and most of the dorsum of the foot and toes except

Figure 9-1. *The distal sensory branches of the superficial peroneal nerve.*

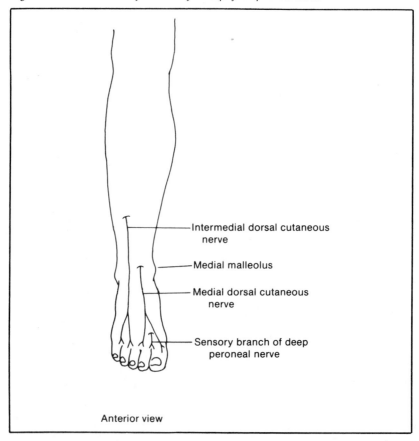

Intermedial dorsal cutaneous nerve

Medial malleolus

Medial dorsal cutaneous nerve

Sensory branch of deep peroneal nerve

Anterior view

the first dorsal web space which is innervated by the deep peroneal nerve. The peroneus longus and peroneus brevis receive their motor innervation from proximal branches of the superficial peroneal nerve.

Applications

Study of the superficial peroneal nerve is useful in distinguishing L_5 radiculopathies from more distal lesions involving the peroneal fibers.

Procedure

1. Recording electrode placement
   a. Plantar-flex and invert the foot and palpate the superficial peroneal nerve (intermediate dorsal cutaneous branch) over the dorsum of the foot medial to the lateral malleolus (Fig. 9-1).
   b. Place the G_1 active recording electrode directly over the nerve about one finger-breadth medial to the lateral malleolus (Fig. 9-2).
   c. Place the G_2 reference electrode 3 to 4 cm distal to the G_1 electrode.
2. Ground is placed close to the recording electrode.
3. Stimulate 12 cm proximal to the G_1 electrode along the anterolateral surface of the distal leg.

Normal values are listed in Table 9-1.

Figure 9-2. *Electrode placement for antidromic recording of the sensory response from the superficial peroneal nerve.*

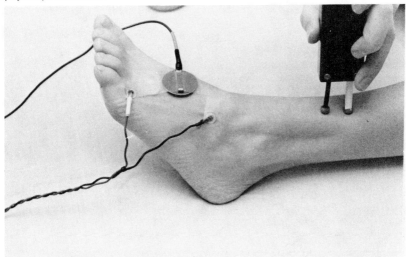

Table 9-1. *Normal Values: Superficial Peroneal Nerve*

Parameter	Lower leg to ankle	Reference
Amplitude (μV) (peak to peak)	>5	[2]
Peak latency (msec) (distance 12 cm)	2.9 ± 0.3 (<3.5)	[1]
Maximum conduction velocity (m/sec)	53.3 ± 5.7 (40–68)	[3]

References

1. Jabre, J. F. The superficial peroneal sensory nerve revisited. *Arch. Neurol.* 38:666, 1981.
2. Lambert, E. H., and Daube, J. R. (Chairmen). *Special Course #16: Clinical Electromyography.* American Academy of Neurology Meeting, Chicago, Ill., April 23–28, 1979.
3. Ma, D. M., and Liveson, J. A. *Nerve Conduction Handbook.* Philadelphia: Davis, 1983.

Tibial Nerve 10
Motor and Sensory Studies

Anatomy
The *tibial nerve* is composed of fibers from the $L_{4,5}$ and $S_{1,2,3}$ roots. The tibial nerve descends deep in the leg to the medial aspect of the ankle, where it travels under the flexor retinaculum (tarsal tunnel) behind the medial malleolus. In the distal end of the tarsal tunnel it bifurcates into the medial and lateral plantar nerves. The medial branch innervates the medial foot muscles including the abductor hallucis, and the lateral branch innervates the lateral foot muscles including the abductor digiti quinti (Fig. 10-1). The sensory innervation is analogous to the hand with the medial plantar nerve supplying the skin over the medial three and a half toes and the lateral plantar nerve supplying the skin over the lateral one and a half toes. The tibial nerve provides motor innervation to the muscles of the posterior compartment of the calf and the foot and sensory innervation to the skin of the heel and sole.

Applications
The tibial nerve may be compromised in the popliteal fossa (e.g., by trauma, a popliteal aneurysm or a synovial cyst). The *tarsal tunnel syndrome* is an entrapment of the nerve under the flexor retinaculum at the ankle behind the medial malleolus. In the tarsal tunnel the trunk of the tibial nerve may be compromised or either of its two branches may be affected separately.

Procedure
Motor

1. Recording electrode placement
   a. There are two alternatives:
      (1) G_1 recording electrode over the abductor hallucis (AH) to test the medial plantar branch (Fig. 10-2).
      (2) G_1 recording electrode over the abductor digiti quinti (ADQ) to test the lateral plantar branch (see Fig. 7-3).
   b. G_2 recording electrode over the great toe for method (1) or over the fifth toe for method (2).

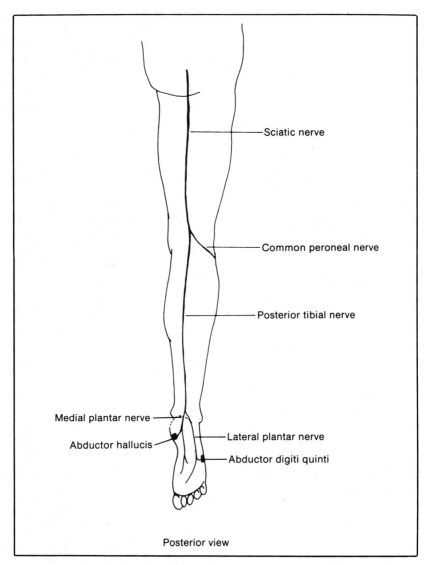

Figure 10-1. Origin and course of the posterior tibial nerve.

2. Ground is placed close to the recording electrodes.
3. Stimulation
    a. Middle of the popliteal crease (see Fig. 7-5).
    b. Slightly posterior to the medial malleolus, 10 cm proximal to the G_1 electrode (Fig. 10-2). Both plantar branches are stimulated at this point.
4. Distance measurement to the ADQ should be with an obstetric caliper whereas a tape measure can be used for the measurement to the AH.

Normal values are listed in Table 10-1.

Plantar Nerves: Mixed Nerves (Orthodromic)
The medial and lateral plantar nerves can be stimulated with ring electrodes placed on the first and fifth toes respectively, but the sensory responses are generally very small and are often difficult to elicit even in normals. Mixed nerve responses are technically easier to elicit and are larger in amplitude [6].

1. Recording electrode placement (Fig. 10-3): Bipolar electrode just posterior and proximal to the medial malleolus.
2. Ground is placed between stimulating and recording electrodes.
3. Stimulation
    a. Medial plantar nerve: 14 cm proximal to G_1, on the sole of the foot, in line with the first toe interspace (Fig. 10-3).

Figure 10-2. *Electrode placement for recording from the abductor hallucis and the distal stimulation site for the tibial nerve.*

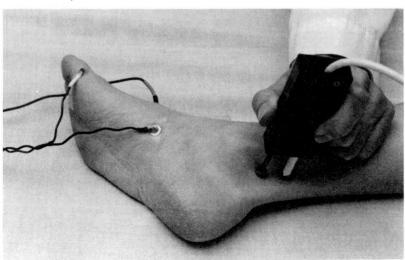

Table 10-1. *Normal Values: Tibial Motor*

Segment	Latency (msec) or NCV (m/sec)	Amplitude peak to peak (mV)	Reference
Ankle to abductor hallucis		19.1 ± 7.2 (>5 mV)	[4]
Ankle to abductor hallucis (distance 10 cm)	3.9 ± 0.6 (2.7–5.1)		[1,5]
Ankle to abductor hallucis R-L latency difference	<1.8		[3]
Ankle to ADQ (distance 10 cm, measured with caliper)	4.5 ± 0.7 (<5.8)		[1]
Popliteal fossa* to gastrocnemius (distance 18 cm)	4.7 ± 0.4 (3.9–5.5)		[5]
Popliteal fossa to ankle	49.0 ± 3.0 (43–55)		[2,5]

ADQ = abductor digiti quinti.
* Concentric needle recording.

Figure 10-3. *Electrode placement for plantar nerve stimulation. (S_1 = medial plantar nerve stimulation; S_2 = lateral plantar nerve stimulation; G_1 and G_2 = recording electrodes over the tibial nerve at the ankle; G_0 = ground.)*

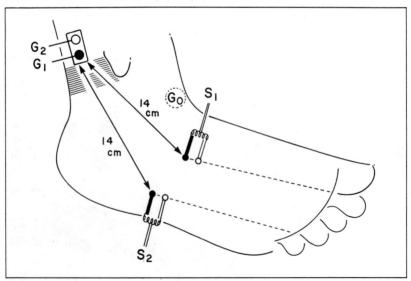

Table 10-2. *Normal Values: Plantar Orthodromic*

Parameter	Medial plantar nerve	Lateral plantar nerve
Amplitude (μV) (peak to peak)	10–30	8–20
Peak latency (msec) (distance 14 cm)	3.2 ± 0.26 (2.6–3.7)	3.2 ± 0.25 (2.7–3.7)

Source: Values from M. A. Saeed and P. Gaetens [6].

    b. Lateral plantar nerve: 14 cm proximal to G_1, on the sole of the foot, in line with the fourth toe interspace (Fig. 10-3).
4. Distances measured with a flexible tape measure.

Normal values are listed in Table 10-2.

References
1. Fu, R., DeLisa, J. A., and Kraft, G. H.   Motor nerve latencies through the tarsal tunnel in normal adult subjects: Standard determination corrected for temperature and distance. *Arch. Phys. Med. Rehabil.* 61:243, 1980.
2. Jiminez, J., Easton, J. K. M., and Redford, J. B.   Conduction studies of anterior and posterior tibial nerves. *Arch. Phys. Med. Rehabil.* 51:164, 1970.
3. Kimura, J.   *Electrodiagnosis in Diseases of Nerve and Muscle: Principles and Practice.* Philadelphia: Davis, 1984.
4. Oh, S. J.   *Clinical Electromyography: Nerve Conduction Studies.* Baltimore: University Park Press, 1984.
5. Rigshospitalet Laboratory of Clinical Neurophysiology. *Electromyography: Sensory and Motor Conduction: Findings in Normal Subjects.* Copenhagen: Rigshospitalet, 1975.
6. Saeed, M. A., Gaetens, P.   Compound nerve action potentials of the medial and lateral plantar nerves through the tarsal tunnel. *Arch. Phys. Med. Rehabil.* 63:304, 1982.

Sural Nerve **11**
Sensory Studies

Anatomy

The *sural nerve* is formed by the union of the medial sural cutaneous branch of the tibial nerve and the lateral sural cutaneous branch of the peroneal nerve. Sural sensory fibers originate from the S_1 root and traverse the sacral plexus and sciatic nerve. The sural nerve becomes superficial at approximately the junction of the middle and lower third of the calf, then descends slightly lateral to the Achilles tendon. It passes behind the lateral malleolus and terminates as the *lateral dorsal cutaneous nerve* over the lateral side of the foot (Fig. 11-1).

Figure 11-1. *Origin and course of the sural nerve.*

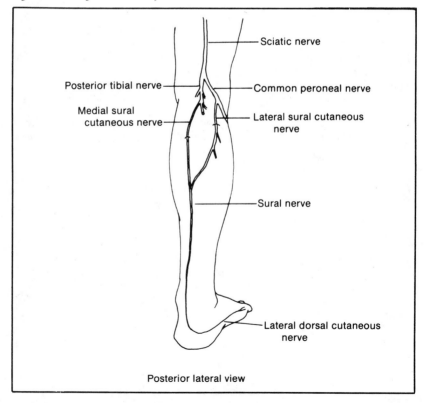

Sciatic nerve

Posterior tibial nerve

Common peroneal nerve

Medial sural cutaneous nerve

Lateral sural cutaneous nerve

Sural nerve

Lateral dorsal cutaneous nerve

Posterior lateral view

Applications

Study of the sural nerve is useful in distinguishing S_1 radiculopathies from lesions distal to the S_1 dorsal root ganglion. The sural nerve often develops abnormal responses—most commonly, amplitude decrement early in the course of polyneuropathies. It may be difficult to evoke a

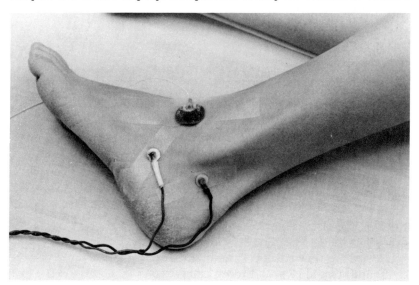

Figure 11-2. *Recording electrode placement for the sural nerve.*

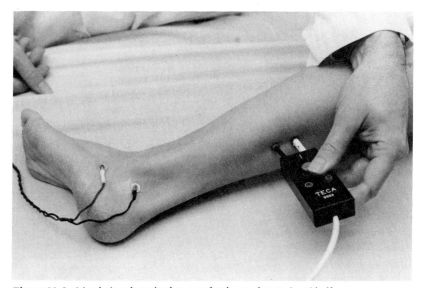

Figure 11-3. *Stimulating electrode placement for the sural nerve in midcalf.*

Table 11-1. Normal Values: Sural Antidromic Sensory

Parameter	Calf to ankle	Reference
Amplitude (μV) (peak to peak)	16.6 ± 7.5 (5–56)	[2]
Maximum conduction velocity (m/sec)	46.2 ± 3.3 (40.0–59.3)	[1]
Peak latency (msec) (distance 14 cm)	3.6 ± 0.4 (2.8–4.4)	[2]
Peak conduction velocity (m/sec)	43.3 ± 4.3 (>34.7)	[3]

sural sensory nerve action potential in normal persons over 60 years of age.

Procedure
Antidromic Sensory

1. Recording electrode placement
   a. Place the G_1 electrode behind the lateral malleolus (Fig. 11-2).
   b. Place the G_2 electrode 3 cm distal to the G_1 electrode.
2. Ground: placed close to the recording electrode.
3. Stimulate with the cathode located in the midcalf, 14 cm proximal to the G_1 recording electrode (Fig. 11-3).

Normal values are listed in Table 11-1.

References
1. DiBenedetto, M.   Sensory nerve conduction in lower extremities. *Arch. Phys. Med. Rehabil.* 51:253, 1970.
2. Izzo, K. L., et al.   Sensory conduction studies of the branches of the superficial peroneal nerve. *Arch. Phys. Med. Rehabil.* 62:24, 1981.
3. Oh, S. J.   *Clinical Electromyography: Nerve Conduction Studies.* Baltimore: University Park Press, 1984.

Femoral Nerve *12*
Motor Studies

Anatomy

Receiving fibers from L$_{2,3,4}$, the femoral nerve is the largest branch of the lumbar plexus. About 4 to 5 cm below the inguinal ligament the femoral nerve breaks up into several branches, the largest and longest of which is the saphenous nerve which provides sensory innervation to

Figure 12-1. *Origin and course of the femoral nerve.*

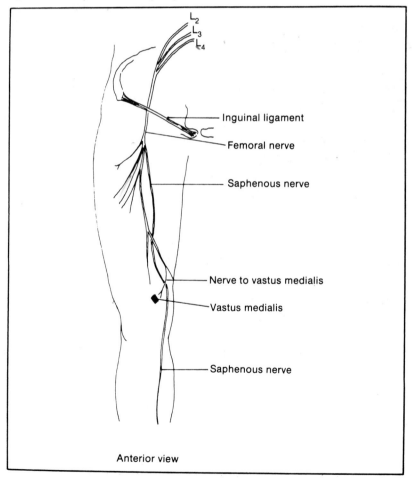

Anterior view

the medial aspect of the lower leg and foot (Fig. 12-1). The femoral nerve supplies motor innervation to the iliacus, pectineus, sartorius, and quadriceps femoris muscles and sensory innervation to the anterolateral thigh. The quadriceps femoris consists of the rectus femoris, vastus lateralis, vastus medialis, and vastus intermedius. The muscle fibers in all these muscles except the vastus intermedius run obliquely (Fig. 12-2) so the motor endplate zones (concentrated in the middle of muscle fibers) form vertical bands [1]. This arrangement of motor endplates enables the conduction velocity to be calculated between two recording points within the muscle. The vastus medialis and rectus femoris muscles are commonly used in motor conduction studies of the femoral nerve (Fig. 12-3).

Applications

Ischemic femoral mononeuropathy due to small vessel disease is commonly seen in diabetic patients. Compression or injury of the nerve within the pelvis has been reported with retroperitoneal hematoma,

Figure 12-2. *Quadriceps femoris muscle and the stimulation point at Hunter's canal.*

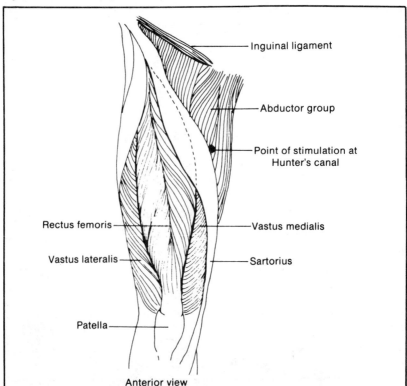

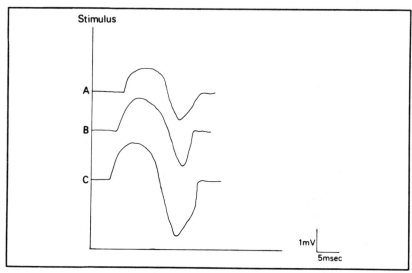

Figure 12-3. *Motor response from the vastus medialis with stimulation above the inguinal ligament (A), below the inguinal ligament (B), and at Hunter's canal (C).*

tumors, and pelvic fractures. A prolonged dorsal lithotomy position can result in compression at the level of the inguinal ligament [3]. Femoral conduction velocity and distal latencies are often impaired in demyelinating neuropathies [1].

Procedure
Motor

1. Recording electrode placement: Monopolar (Fig. 12-4) or concentric needle recording electrodes can be used. With monopolar recording:

Figure 12-4. *Electrode placement for recording from the vastus medialis and stimulation of the femoral nerve at Hunter's canal.*

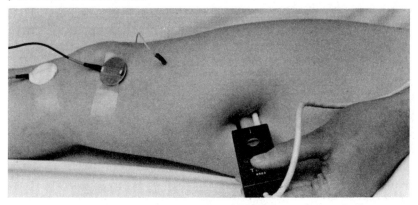

a. The G_1 needle electrode is placed in the vastus medialis (Fig. 12-4).

b. The G_2 surface disc electrode is placed over the proximal tibia.

2. Ground is placed close to the recording electrodes.

3. Stimulation

   a. Percutaneous

      (1) Just proximal to the inguinal ligament over the projected course of the femoral nerve (Fig. 12-5).

      (2) Just distal to the inguinal ligament, lateral to the palpable femoral artery (Fig. 12-6).

      (3) At Hunter's canal along the medial aspect of the thigh. Hunter's canal is deep to the sartorius muscle along the middle third of the thigh (see Figs. 12-2 and 12-4).

      Pitfalls: Unintentional submaximal stimulation with the percutaneous technique which can result in latencies that are unusually prolonged. An H-reflex with a latency of 14 to 17 msec is sometimes elicited with submaximal stimulation [1,2].

   b. Transcutaneous stimulation causes less discomfort, especially in obese patients. The cathode is a monopolar EMG needle and the anode is a surface disc electrode placed over the nearby skin. As the needle tip approaches the femoral nerve the vastus medialis can be observed to contract, thus making it possible to avoid insertion directly into the nerve [4]. Transcutaneous stimulation is especially useful at Hunter's canal.

Normal values are listed in Table 12-1.

Figure 12-5. *Stimulation of the femoral nerve proximal to the inguinal ligament.*

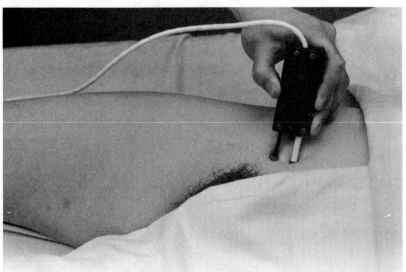

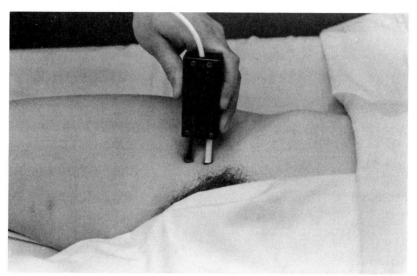

Figure 12-6. *Stimulation of the femoral nerve distal to the inguinal ligament.*

Table 12-1. *Normal Values: Femoral Motor*

	Mean	SD	Range
Distance from above inguinal ligament to vastus medialis	35.2 cm	1.9 cm	29–38 cm
Latency from above inguinal ligament to vastus medialis	7.1 msec	0.7 msec	6.1–8.4 msec
Latency from below inguinal ligament to vastus medialis	6.0 msec	0.7 msec	5.5–7.5 msec
Latency from Hunter's canal to vastus medialis	4.0 msec	—	—
NCV from above inguinal ligament to Hunter's canal	66.7 m/sec	7.4 m/sec	50–96 m/sec
NCV from below inguinal ligament to Hunter's canal	69.4 m/sec	9.2 m/sec	50–90 m/sec
Distance across inguinal ligament	5.5 cm	1.6 cm	4.2–6.6 cm
Delay across inguinal ligament	1.2 msec	0.4 msec	0.8–1.8 msec

Source: Values from Johnson [2].

Table 12-2. *Normal Values: Femoral Nerve Conduction Velocity (NCV) between Two Recording Sites*

Parameters	Inguinal region to rectus femoris	Reference
Latency at 14 cm	3.3 ± 0.36 (2.6–4.2)	[5]
Latency at 28 cm	5.5 ± 0.47 (4.7–6.7)	[5]
NCV between the recording sites	64.3 ± 8.00 (50.0–79.4)	[5]

Source: Values from Schubert [5].

Nerve Conduction Velocity Between Two Recording Sites
Nerve conduction velocity (NCV) can also be calculated between two recording sites in the intramuscular nerve fibers (Table 12-2) [1,5].

References
1. Gassel, M. M.   A study of femoral nerve conduction: An aid in differentiating neuritis of the femoral nerve from other causes of proximal neurogenic and muscular disease. *Arch. Neurol.* 9:607, 1963.
2. Johnson, E. W., Wood, D. K., and Powers, J. J.   Femoral nerve conduction studies. *Arch. Phys. Med. Rehabil.* 49:528, 1968.
3. Kopell, P., and Thompson, W. A. L.   Peripheral Entrapment Neuropathies. Baltimore: Williams & Wilkins, 1963.
4. Lambert, E. H., and Daube, J. R. (Chairmen).   *Special Course #16: Clinical Electromyography.* American Academy of Neurology Meeting, Chicago, Ill, Apr. 23–28, 1979.
5. Schubert, H. A., and Keil, E. W.   Femoral nerve conduction velocity. *Am. J. Phys. Med.* 47:302, 1968.

Saphenous Nerve 13
Sensory Studies

Anatomy
The *saphenous nerve* ($L_{3,4}$) is the largest and longest division of the femoral nerve originating just distal to the inguinal ligament. The saphenous nerve descends deep to the sartorius within the adductor canal (*Hunter's canal*) in the medial thigh and exits from it about 10 cm above the medial epicondyle of the femur. It runs down the leg just behind the medial border of the tibial bone. Approximately 7 cm in front of the ankle it passes in front of the medial malleolus and finally terminates on the dorsum of the foot (Fig. 13-1). The saphenous nerve provides cutaneous innervation to the medial leg and foot.

Applications
Study of the saphenous nerve is useful in distinguishing L_3 and L_4 radiculopathies from lesions distal to the L_3 and L_4 dorsal root ganglia involving the lumbar plexus, femoral nerve, or saphenous nerve. Injury to the saphenous nerve can occur with knee surgery, vascular surgery, and venous stripping [1]. Entrapment is described at the exit from the Hunter's canal [1] and between the sartorius and gracilis tendons at the knee [2].

Procedure
Antidromic Sensory

1. Recording electrode placement
   a. Place the G_1 recording electrode between the medial malleolus and the tibialis anterior tendon at the ankle (Fig. 13-2).
   b. Place the G_2 recording electrode 3 cm distal to the G_2 electrode.
2. Ground is placed close to the recording electrodes (Fig. 13-2).
3. Stimulate the saphenous nerve deep to the medial border of the tibia, 14 cm proximal to G_1. The stimulating electrodes must be pushed in firmly between the medial belly of the gastrocnemius and the tibia.

Normal values are listed in Table 13-1.

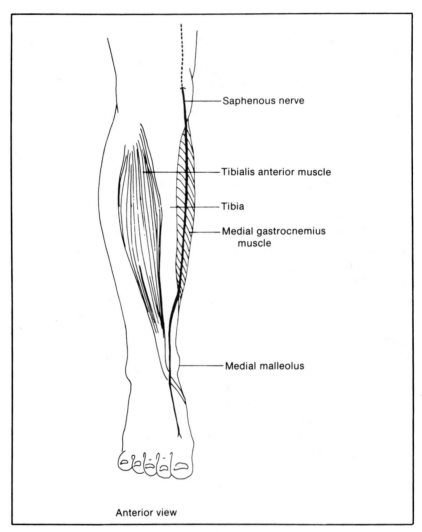

Figure 13-1. *Distal superficial course of the saphenous nerve.*

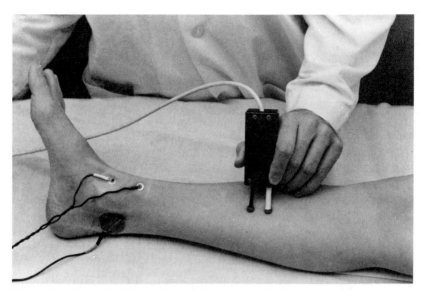

Figure 13-2. Electrode placement for antidromic recording of the saphenous nerve sensory response.

Table 13-1. Normal Values: Saphenous Antidromic Sensory

Parameter	Peak latency (msec)	Amplitude peak to peak (μV)	Peak NCV (m/sec)	Reference
Lower leg to ankle (14 cm)	3.6 ± 0.4 (<4.4)	9.0 ± 3.4 (<5 in 1/3)	41.7 ± 3.4 (>35)	[3]

References

1. Dawson, D. M., Hallet, M., Millender, L. H. *Entrapment Neuropathies.* Boston: Little, Brown, 1983.
2. Ma, D. M., and Liveson, J. A. *Nerve Conduction Handbook.* Philadelphia: Davis, 1983.
3. Wainapel, S. F., Kim, D. J., and Ebel, A. Conduction studies of the saphenous nerve in healthy subjects. *Arch. Phys. Med. Rehabil.* 59:316, 1978.

Facial Nerve 14
Direct Stimulation and Blink Reflex

Anatomy
The *facial nerve* emerges from the skull at the stylomastoid foramen (Fig. 14-1) and gives off five main branches (temporal, zygomatic, buccal, mandibular, and cervical) just anterior and inferior to the tragus of the ear. The motor division of the facial nerve innervates the facial muscles, platysma, and a few muscles behind the ear (Fig. 14-2).

Applications
Facial nerve palsy is the most common cranial mononeuropathy, and most of these cases are idiopathic (e.g., Bell's palsy). Complete recovery occurs in over half the patients, but 5 to 10 percent have significant sequelae [6].

Other less common causes of facial paralysis are trauma, middle ear infection, geniculate herpes zoster (Ramsay Hunt syndrome), Lyme disease, diabetic ischemic mononeuropathy, and cerebellopontine angle tumors. Bilateral facial paralysis can be seen with acquired demyelinating neuropathy (Guillain-Barré syndrome), sarcoidosis, and leptomeningeal carcinomatosis.

Facial nerve conduction studies done 5 to 7 days after the onset of

Figure 14-1. *Facial nerve in relationship to the mastoid process of the temporal bone.*

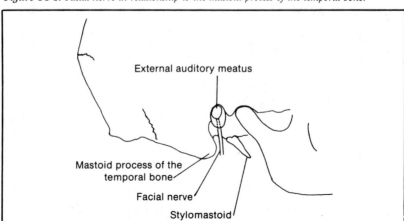

External auditory meatus

Mastoid process of the
temporal bone

Facial nerve

Stylomastoid

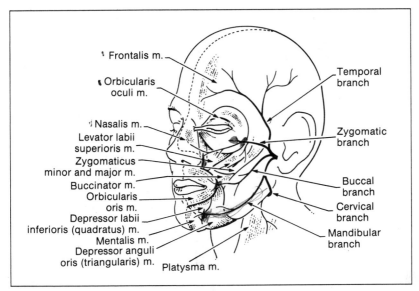

Figure 14-2. *Facial nerve branches and innervation.*

paralysis are commonly performed in patients with Bell's palsy and provide useful prognostic information [5,6]. Comparison with the non-paretic side is more useful than the absolute values. A greater than 50 to 70 percent reduction in amplitude is the single most important criterion. Latency prolongation of greater than 25 percent relative to the nonparetic side is also significant [6]. Other criteria are as follows.

1. Normal results: Complete recovery within 2 months.
2. Reduced amplitude (10 to 30 percent of normal side): Usually good recovery over 2 to 8 months, but mild to moderate chance of sequelae.
3. Reduced amplitude less than 10 percent of nonparetic side or no response: High incidence of aberrant regeneration with facial synkinesis or crocodile-tear phenomenon. Most patients will have satisfactory recovery of function over 6 to 12 months, but a few patients in this group may have no functional recovery and develop a contracture.

Facial nerve repetitive stimulation is useful for evaluating proximal muscles for decrement in patients suspected of having myasthenia gravis.

Procedure
The procedure described below is for surface recording from the nasalis muscle. Motor responses from other muscles such as the mentalis, trian-

gularis, orbicularis oris, orbicularis oculi, and frontalis (Fig. 14-2) often require the use of needles for recording. Monopolar needles with a surface disc reference on the opposite side of the face provide the most consistent results from these muscles [6].

1. Recording electrode placement (Fig. 14-3)
    a. G_1 disc electrode is placed over the nasalis muscle 1 to 2 cm above the external naris (Fig. 14-3).
    b. G_2 electrode is placed in the same position on the opposite side of the face.
2. Ground is placed on the chin.
3. Stimulate with a hand-held bipolar surface prong.
    a. Place the cathode near the stylomastoid foramen just below and

Figure 14-3. *Recording electrode placement for left facial nerve stimulation. Active (G_1) electrode (black wire) is over the ipsilateral nasalis muscle; G_2 electrode (marked with white tape) is over the contralateral nasalis; ground is under the chin.*

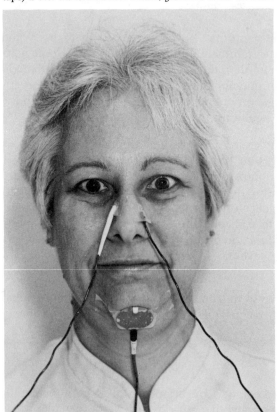

anterior to the tip of the mastoid beneath the earlobe. The anode should be inferior to the cathode and may need to be rotated to reduce artifact or eliminate masseter contraction (Fig. 14-4).

b. If method (A) fails, the cathode can be placed just anterior and inferior to the tragus of the earlobe (Fig. 14-5).

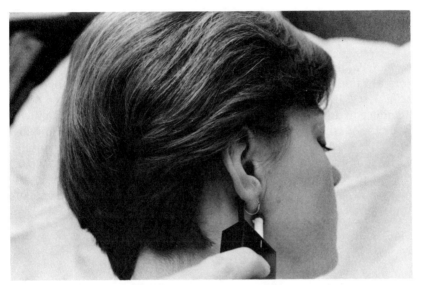

Figure 14-4. *Facial nerve stimulation near the stylomastoid foramen.*

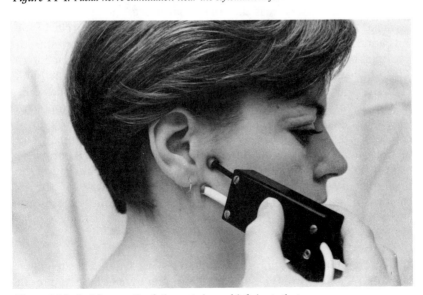

Figure 14-5. *Facial nerve stimulation anterior and inferior to the tragus.*

Table 14-1. *Normal Values: Postauricular Stimulation of the Facial Nerve*

Muscle	Onset latency (msec)	Reference
Nasalis (8.8–13.1 cm)[a]	3.5 ± 0.4 (<4.2)	[5]
Triangularis (7–13 cm)[b]	3.2 ± 0.4 (<4.1)	[6]
Orbicularis oris (9.9–15.5 cm)[b]	3.8 ± 0.8 (<4.8)	[6]
Frontalis (12.5–18 cm)[b]	4.5 ± 0.5 (<5.5)	[6]

[a] Surface disc recording.
[b] Needle recording.

Normal Values

Normal values must always be compared with those from the opposite facial nerve. Peak-to-peak amplitudes are generally 1 to 4 mV [4,6]; a difference in amplitude of greater than 50 percent and a latency difference of more than 25 percent, or 0.6 msec, represents a significant abnormality [4,6]. The distance from the cathode to the active recording electrode must be identical on the two sides. An increase in distance of 1 cm between the stimulating and recording electrodes results in an increase in latency of 0.23 msec [6]. Normal values for postauricular stimulation of the facial nerve are listed in Table 14-1.

Blink Reflex

Anatomy

The blink reflex is analogous to the clinically elicited corneal reflex. The afferent limb of the reflex is the trigeminal nerve; the efferent limb is the facial nerve; and synaptic connections between them occur in the pons and lateral medulla (Fig. 14-6A). Electrical stimulation of the supraorbital branch of the trigeminal nerve results in reflex contraction of both orbicularis oculi muscles. However, EMG recordings of the blink reflex show two separate components: an early R_1 component seen only ipsilaterally on the side of the stimulation and a late R_2 component recorded bilaterally [3] (Fig. 14-6). The R_1 component is thought to represent a disynaptic pathway between the main sensory nucleus of the trigeminal nerve and the ipsilateral facial nucleus. The R_2 probably results from polysynaptic connections between the spinal nucleus of the trigeminal nerve and bilateral facial nuclei [1] (Fig. 14-6A). The R_1 latency is relatively constant, whereas the R_2 response has a more variable latency and tends to habituate with repeated stimulation.

Applications

Figure 14-6B illustrates abnormalities with lesions at different sites along the blink reflex pathway. Lesions involving the trigeminal nerve result

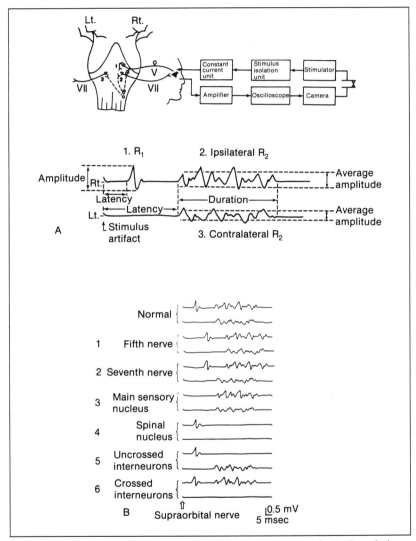

Figure 14-6. *Blink reflex. A. Pathway for R_1 through the pons (1) and for R_2 through the pons and lateral medulla (2 and 3). B. Blink reflex abnormalities with lesions at different sites along the reflex pathway. (From J. Kimura.* Electrodiagnosis in Disease of Nerve and Muscle: Technique and Interpretation. *Philadelphia: Davis, 1983. Used by permission.)*

in delayed latencies bilaterally, or there may be a total absence of responses on stimulation of the affected trigeminal nerve. Patients with idiopathic trigeminal neuralgia usually have normal blink reflexes.

In contrast, facial nerve lesions result in unilateral delayed latencies or absent responses on the clinically affected side, regardless of the side of stimulation. The blink reflex evaluates proximal and distal conduction and is more sensitive than direct facial nerve stimulation in demonstrating facial nerve abnormalities.

The blink reflex is particularly sensitive as a screening test for suspected cerebellopontine angle tumors such as acoustic neuromas, 85 percent of which have an abnormal blink reflex [2]. Afferent or efferent fibers can be affected.

The blink reflex may be useful in demonstrating a silent brainstem lesion in patients with multiple sclerosis. The reflex may be abnormal in 40 percent of patients without clinical evidence of a brainstem lesion [1].

Figure 14-7. *Electrode placement for the blink reflex. Active recording electrodes (G_1) are below lateral canthi bilaterally; reference recording electrodes (G_2; marked with white tape) are over the temporal regions bilaterally; ground is under the chin. The supraorbital nerve is stimulated over the medial third of the supraorbital ridge.*

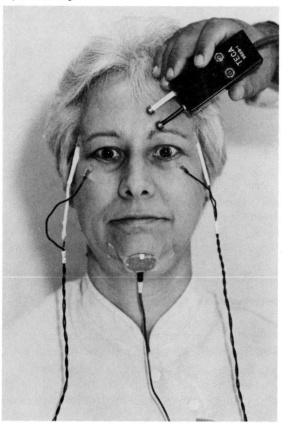

Table 14-2. *Normal Values: Blink Reflex*

Parameter	Latency (msec) mean ± SD (normal limit)*	Side-to-side difference (msec) mean ± SD (normal limit)*
R_1 component	10.45 ± 0.84 (<13)	0.3 ± 0.9 (<1.2)
R_2 ipsilateral	30.5 ± 3.4 (<41)	1.0 ± 1.2 (<5)
R_2 contralateral	30.5 ± 4.4 (<44)	1.6 ± 1.7 (<7)

* Normal limit defined as 3 SD from mean.
Source: Values from Kimura [1].

Patients with demyelinating neuropathies (acquired and hereditary) often have abnormal latencies even with relatively little clinical facial weakness [2]. The pattern of abnormalities may be afferent or efferent.

Spread of the blink reflex into muscles other than the orbicularis oculi is seen in facial synkinesis (from aberrant regeneration) and in hemifacial spasm (from ephaptic transmission).

Procedure

The machine settings for the blink reflex are given in Appendix I.
1. Recording electrode placement (Fig. 14-7)
   a. Place G_1 active electrodes bilaterally on the skin over the orbicularis oculi muscle just below the lateral canthi (Fig. 14-7). Two channels are necessary for simultaneous recording from both sides.
   b. Place G_2 reference electrodes on the temple or lateral nose.
2. Ground is placed on the chin.
3. Stimulation
   a. Electrical: Stimulate the supraorbital nerve over a palpable groove at the medial third of the supraorbital ridge (Fig. 14-7). An initial stimulus duration of 0.05 msec and a stimulus frequency of 0.2 Hz (see Appendix I) is optimal.
   b. Mechanical: a glabellar tap with a special hammer that triggers the sweep can also be used to elicit a blink reflex. However, in this case bilateral R_1 responses are seen.
4. Measurement: The shortest latency from the stimulus onset to the initial baseline deflection of the R_1 and R_2 components in a series of about ten responses is used.

Normal values are listed in Table 14-2.

References
1. Kimura, J.   Electrically elicited blink reflex in multiple sclerosis: Review of 260 patients over a seven-year period. *Brain* 98:413, 1975.
2. Kimura, J.   *Electrodiagnosis in Disease of Nerve and Muscle: Technique and Interpretation*. Philadelphia: Davis, 1983.
3. Kimura, J., Power J. M., and Van Allen, M. W.   Reflex response of orbicularis muscle to supraorbital nerve stimulation: Study in normal subjects and peripheral facial palsies. *Arch. Neurol.* 21:193, 1969.
4. Lambert, E. H., and Daube, J. R. (Chairmen):   *Special Course #16: Clinical Electromyography*. American Academy of Neurology Meeting, Chicago, Ill., April 23–28, 1979.
5. Miller, D. W., Nelson, J. A., and Bender, L. F.   Measurement of latency in facial nerve in normal and uremic persons. *Arch. Phys. Med. Rehabil.* 51:413, 1970.
6. Olsen, P. Z.   Prediction of recovery in Bell's palsy. *Acta. Neurol. Scand.* (Suppl. 61) 52:1, 1975.

The F-Wave 15

Anatomy and Physiology

The *F-wave* is a late compound muscle action potential resulting from the backfiring of antidromically activated motor neurons, which can be recorded with a supramaximal electrical stimulus from almost every skeletal muscle [3,5,9]. It was so named because it was initially recorded in the foot muscles [8]. Electrical stimulation of motor fibers results in an impulse that travels both orthodromically toward the muscle and antidromically toward the spinal cord. The short latency direct response from orthodromic conduction is called the M-wave, and the late response occurring after the M-wave is termed the F-wave. With more proximal stimulation the M-latency increases whereas the F-latency decreases (Fig. 15-1), clearly indicating that the impulse for the F-wave initially travels antidromically. The latency of an F-wave includes the time required for the evoked action potential to ascend antidromically to the anterior horn cells, the delay time in the anterior horn cells (1 msec), and the time required for the resultant action potential to descend orthodromically from the anterior horn cell to the muscle fibers [3]. F-responses vary in latency, configuration, and amplitude with repeated stimuli (Fig. 15-1) because different groups of motor neurons are activated with each stimulus. The *shortest latency* in a series of recorded F-waves (Fig. 15-2) is a measure of the fastest conducting fibers and is the parameter generally used, although some investigators recommend using the average latency [2]. The percentage of stimuli that elicits an F-response is termed *F-persistence* and is normally 90 to 100 percent [1]. Impersistence of F-waves (Fig. 15-2) may be an early sign of a neuropathy.

F-wave conduction velocity calculations have been used [4] but the inaccuracies in distance measurements can add significant errors in converting F-latency to F-wave conduction velocity [11]. The normal parameters of the F-wave are summarized below:

Threshold	Seen with supramaximal stimulation.
Latency	The minimal–maximal latency difference (chronodispersion) is normally a few milliseconds. The latency increases with more distal sites.
Amplitude	1 to 5 percent of M-wave.
Configuration	Variable; triphasic to polyphasic.

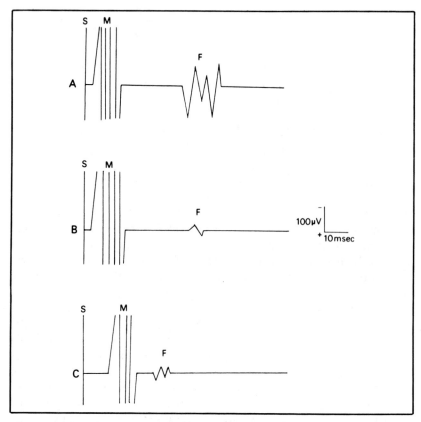

Figure 15-1. *F-wave with distal (A and B) and proximal (C) stimulation of the same nerve. Note variation of latency, amplitude, and configuration in A and B; more proximal stimulation results in a shorter F-wave latency (C). Stimulus (S) and M-response (M) are off the vertical scale.*

Applications

Measurements of F-wave latencies supplement routine nerve conduction studies since they also evaluate the proximal conduction in motor fibers. They are of value in disorders involving the nerve roots, plexuses, and the proximal segments of peripheral nerves. The determination of F-wave latencies is particularly valuable in evaluating patients with demyelinating polyradiculoneuropathies.

Procedure

The recommended machine settings are given in Appendix I.

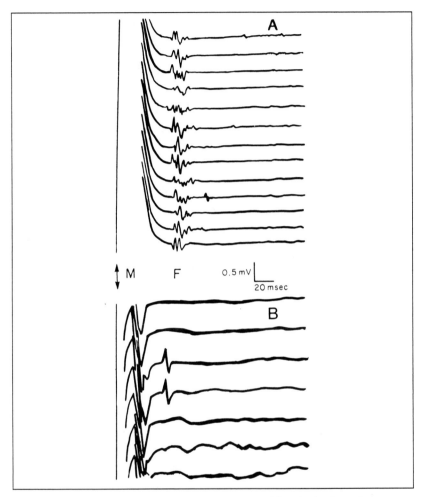

Figure 15-2. *Tibial nerve F-waves. Normal (A) occurring with each stimulus and impersistent (B) recorded only twice in this series from a patient with Guillain-Barré syndrome. (M = direct motor response; F = F-wave; arrow indicates point of stimulation.)*

1. Recording electrode placement is the same as for routine motor nerve conduction studies for individual nerves.
2. Stimulation: With the cathode *proximal* to the anode, apply a supra-maximal stimulus to the distal median, ulnar, peroneal, or tibial nerves using the standard electrode placements (Fig. 15-3). More proximal stimulation can also be used with shortening of the F-wave latency.
3. Latency measurement: Ten or more F-waves are recorded (see Fig.

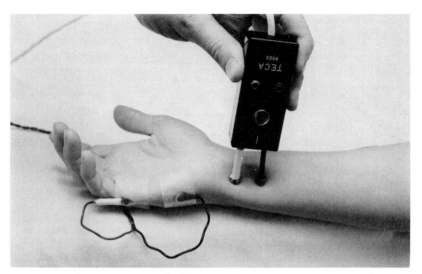

Figure 15-3. *Electrode placement for F-wave determination with ulnar nerve stimulation. Note that the cathode is* **proximal** *to the anode.*

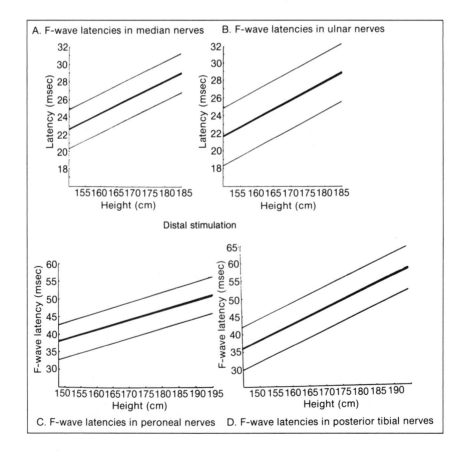

Table 15-1. *Normal Values: F-Response*

Nerve (distal site)	Mean (msec)	Range (msec)	Distance (cm)	Contralateral difference (msec)
Ulnar/hypothenar	26.6	21–32	50–76	0–3
Median/thenar	26.4	22–31	57–73	0–3
Tibial/abductor hallucis brevis	48.6	41–57	106–125	0–4
Peroneal/extensor digitorum brevis	47.4	38–57	102–128	0–4

Source: Values from Daube [7].

15-2) and the shortest latency is used. The patient's height, arm length (cathode to the C_7 spine), or leg length (cathode to the xiphoid or T_{12} spine) should be used when comparing with values from other laboratories (Table 15-1). Nomograms relating F-latency to the height (Fig. 15-4) are useful in individual cases [6,10].

References

1. Cherington, M.   H-reflex and F-response. *Course A: Basic Nerve Conduction and Electromyography*. Ninth Annual Continuing Education Course. American Association of Electromyography and Electrodiagnosis, Boston, MA, Sept. 24, 1986.
2. Fischer, M. A.   *Minimonograph #13: Physiology and Clinical Use of the F-Response*. American Association of Electromyography and Electrodiagnosis, Rochester, MN, June, 1980.
3. Kimura, J.   Clinical value and limitations of F-wave determinations: A comment. *Muscle Nerve* 1:250, 1978.
4. Kimura, J.   *Electrodiagnosis in Diseases of Nerve and Muscle: Technique and Interpretation*. Philadelphia: Davis, 1983.
5. Kimura, J., et al.   Is the F-wave elicited in a select group of motoneurons? *Muscle Nerve* 7:392, 1984.
6. Lachman, T., Shahani, B. T., and Young, R.   Late responses as aids to diagnosis in peripheral neuropathy. *J. Neurol. Neurosurg. Psychiatry* 43:156, 1980.
7. Lambert, E. H., and Daube, J. R. (Chairmen)   *Special Course #16: Clinical Electromyography*. American Academy of Neurology Meeting, Chicago, Ill., April 23–28, 1979.
8. Magladery, J. W., McDougal, D. B.   Electrophysiological studies of nerve and reflex activity in normal man: Part 1, Identification of certain reflexes in the electromyogram and the conduction velocity of peripheral nerve fibers. *Bull. Johns Hopkins Hosp.* 88:265, 1950.

Figure 15-4. *Normal F-wave latencies with distal stimulation relative to height. Median nerve (A), ulnar nerve (B), peroneal nerve (C), and tibial nerve (D). (Modified from S. Oh.* Clinical Electromyography: Nerve Conduction Studies. *Baltimore: University Park Press, 1984. Reprinted with permission of Aspen Publishers, Inc., © 1984.)*

9. Mayer, R. F., and Feldman, R. G.   Observations on the nature of the F-wave in man. *Neurology (Minneap.)* 17:147, 1967.
10. Oh, S.   Clinical *Electromyography: Nerve Conduction Studies.* Baltimore: University Park Press, 1984.
11. Young, R., and Shahani, B. T.   Clinical value and limitations of F-wave determination. *Muscle Nerve* 1:248, 1978.

The H-Reflex 16

Anatomy and Physiology

The H-reflex is an electrically evoked spinal monosynaptic segmental reflex named after Hoffman, who originally described it in 1918 [4]. A submaximal stimulus activates IA afferents (large myelinated fibers with the lowest threshold for activation) in a mixed nerve, which in turn evokes a monosynaptic reflex contraction in the corresponding myotome (Fig. 16-1). With increasing stimulus intensity, motor fibers in the mixed nerve are also activated with the resulting antidromic motor impulse colliding with the reflex impulse and obliterating it or gener-

Figure 16-1. *Diagrammatic representation of stimulation of the posterior tibial nerve to elicit the H-reflex. Note that the cathode is* **proximal** *to the anode.*

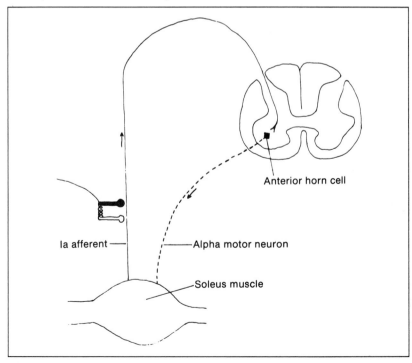

Anterior horn cell

Ia afferent —— —— Alpha motor neuron

—— Soleus muscle

ating an F-wave (Fig. 16-2). The H-reflex amplitude is therefore maximum near the threshold for the M-response and then varies inversely as the M-response amplitude increases with increasing stimulus intensity (Fig. 16-2). The H-reflex latency is similar to that of the F-wave from which it needs to be differentiated. In contrast to the F-wave, the H-reflex has the following characteristics:

1. The stimulus threshold is lower than that required to elicit an M-wave.
2. The latency and waveform tend to be constant at a fixed stimulus intensity since the same motor neurons are activated each time.
3. The amplitude often exceeds that of the M-wave at low stimulus intensity, and the mean amplitude can be 50 to 100 percent of the M-wave [9].
4. The H-reflex is consistently found only in the calf muscles and flexor carpi radialis [5] after the first year of life.

Figure 16-2. *Effect of increasing stimulus strength on H-reflex from subthreshold (1) to supramaximal (8). The H-reflex is usually of maximum amplitude just prior to the appearance of the M-response and then disappears with supramaximal stimulation. (S = stimulus, M = M-response, H = H-reflex).*

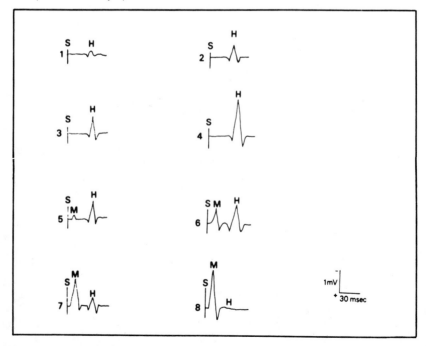

The H-reflex usually has a triphasic configuration with an initial small positivity followed by a large negativity (Fig. 16-2).

Applications

The H-reflex from the soleus is primarily mediated by the S_1 root and is analogous to the ankle jerk, differing only in that the IA afferents are stimulated directly rather than by the stretching of muscle spindles. A unilateral abnormality is therefore helpful in differentiating an S_1 from an L_5 radiculopathy [1].

Bilateral H-reflex abnormalities are a sensitive indicator of a peripheral polyneuropathy (see Fig. 20-4) but need to be differentiated from bilateral S_1 radiculopathies. Sural sensory responses are often abnormal in patients with polyneuropathies but are normal in S_1 radiculopathies. H-reflex abnormalities occur early in the course of demyelinating neuropathies.

H-reflex from the vastus medialis with femoral nerve stimulation [3] and from the extensor digitorum brevis with common peroneal nerve stimulation [2] would be valuable for the evaluation of the L_4 and L_5 roots respectively, but because these H-reflexes are not elicited consistently, they are not clinically useful. In C_6 and C_7 radiculopathies, flexor carpi radialis H-reflex [5] may be prolonged or absent. Unmasking of H-reflexes in muscles in which they are normally not elicited can occur in adults with upper motor neuron lesions.

Procedure

The recommended machine settings are given in Appendix I.

1. Recording electrode placement
   a. The G_1 electrode is placed over the soleus muscle just medial to the tibia, equidistant between the stimulation point and the medial malleolus (Fig. 16-3).
   b. The G_2 electrode is placed over the Achilles tendon.
2. Ground is placed close to the recording electrode.
3. Stimulation: With the stimulating cathode *proximal* to the anode (Fig. 16-4), stimuli just greater than that required to evoke a minimal M-response are applied to the posterior tibial nerve at the center of the popliteal crease. A stimulus of long duration (0.5 to 1.0 msec) with very low intensity is the most suitable. Minimal voluntary plantar flexion can be used to facilitate the response.

4. Latency measurement: The shortest H-wave latency in a series of recordings (Fig. 16-5) is the parameter used. The initial baseline deflection in either direction is used as the point to measure the latency.

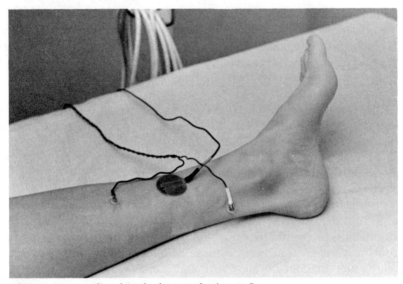

Figure 16-3. *Recording electrode placement for the H-reflex.*

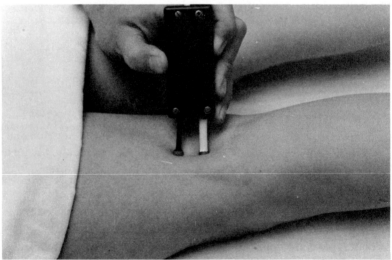

Figure 16-4. *Stimulation of the posterior tibial nerve to elicit the H-reflex. Note that the cathode is **proximal** to the anode.*

Normal Values
The range of the H-reflex latency is 25 to 35 msec with distances of 19 to 25 cm between the stimulating and active recording electrodes [8]. Normal values relative to the height are summarized in Table 16-1.

Nomograms relating the latency to the height (Figs. 16-6, 16-7) are useful in individual cases [1,7].

Figure 16-5. *H-reflex from medial soleus recorded sequentially* (A) *and superimposed* (B). *(M = direct motor response;* H *= H-reflex; the arrow indicates the direction of increasing stimulus intensity.) Note that the topmost trace in the series is an F-wave. The shortest H-reflex in the series is used.*

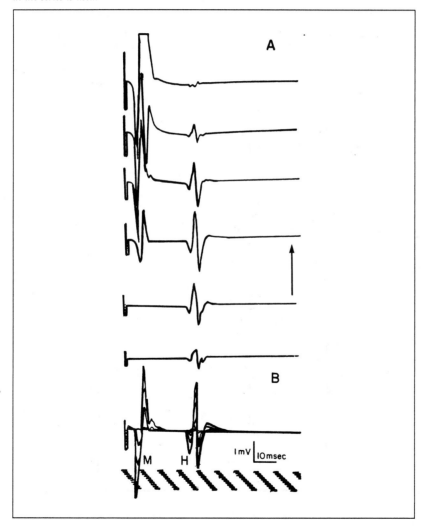

Table 16-1. *Normal Values: H-Reflex*

Reflex	Latency (msec)	R-L latency difference (msec)	Reference
H–Soleus		<1.5	[10]
Short stature (147–160 cm)	28.5 ± 1.8 (<32)		[10]
Median stature (163–175 cm)	29.9 ± 2.1 (<34)		[10]
Tall stature (178–193 cm)	31.5 ± 1.2 (<35)		[10]
H–FCR*	15.9 ± 1.5 (<19)	0.4 ± 0.3 (<1.0)	[5]

* Flexor carpi radialis H-reflex: Stimulate median nerve at elbow and record with surface electrodes. G_1 is placed one-third the distance between the medial epicondyle of the humerus and the radial styloid.

Figure 16-6. *H-reflex latency relative to the leg length (stimulation point to medial malleolus) and age. (From R. I. Braddom and E. W. Johnson. Standardization of H-reflex and diagnostic use in S_1 radiculopathy. Arch. Phys. Med. Rehabil. 55:164, 1974. Used by permission.)*

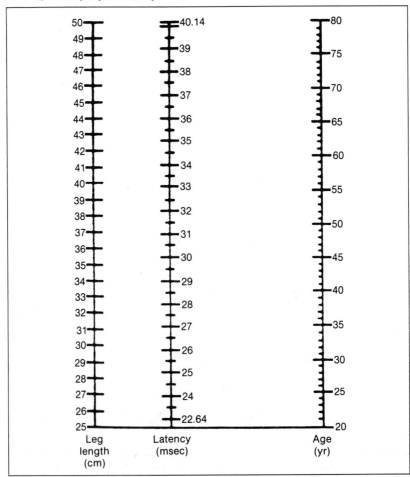

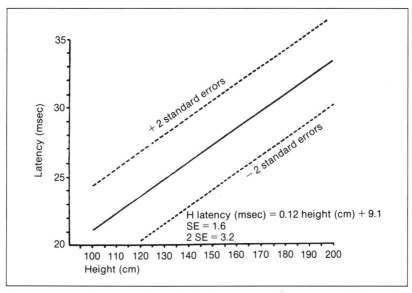

Figure 16-7. *H-reflex latency relative to the height. (From T. Lachman, B. T. Shahani, and R. R. Young. Late responses as aids to diagnosis in peripheral neuropathy.* J. Neurol. Neurosurg. Psychiatry *43:158, 1980. Used by permission.)*

References

1. Braddom, R. I., and Johnson, E. W. Standardization of H-reflex and diagnostic use in S_1 radiculopathy. *Arch. Phys. Med. Rehabil.* 55:161, 1974.

2. Deschuytere, J., and Rosselle, N. Diagnostic use of monosynaptic reflexes in L_5 and S_1 root compression. In J. E. Desmedt (Ed.), *New Developments in Electromyography and Clinical Neurophysiology.* Vol. 3. Basel: Karger, 1973.

3. Gassel, M. M. A study of femoral nerve conduction time: An aid in differentiating neuritis of the femoral nerve from other causes of proximal neurogenic muscular disease. *Arch. Neurol.* 9:607, 1963.

4. Hoffman, P. Uber die Beziehungen der Sehnenreflexe zur willkürlichen Bewegung und zum Tonus. *Z Biol.* 68:351, 1918.

5. Jabre, J. F. Surface recording of the H-reflex of the flexor carpi radialis. *Muscle Nerve* 4:435, 1981.

6. Kraft, G. H., and Johnson, E. W. *Proximal Motor Nerve Conduction and Late Responses.* An AAEE workshop, American Association of Electromyography and Electrodiagnosis, September 1986.

7. Lachman, T., Shahani, B. T., and Young, R. R. Late responses as aids to diagnosis in peripheral neuropathy. *J. Neurol. Neurosurg. Psychiatry* 43:156, 1980.

8. Lambert, E. H., and Daube, J. R. (Chairman). *Special Course #16: Clinical Electromyography.* American Academy of Neurology Meeting, Chicago, Ill., April 23–28, 1979.

9. Shahani, B. T. Late Responses and the "Silent Period". In M. J. Aminoff (Ed.), *Electrodiagnosis in Clinical Neurology.* New York: Churchill Livingstone, 1986.

10. Tonzola, R. F., et al. Usefulness of electrophysiological studies in the diagnosis of lumbosacral root disease. *Ann. Neurol.* 9:305, 1981.

Repetitive Stimulation 17

Repetitive stimulation testing involves repeated supramaximal stimuli given in a short train at a constant frequency to a motor or mixed nerve. The compound motor action potential (CMAP) from a muscle innervated by the stimulated nerve is simultaneously recorded and any changes in the size of the CMAP are measured. It provides an indirect objective assessment of neuromuscular transmission. An understanding of the morphology and physiology is essential to interpret the responses.

Anatomy and Physiology [3,4,5]

The acetylcholine (Ach) in the motor nerve terminal at the neuromuscular junction is stored as vesicles (quanta) in three compartments: (1) immediately available store, (2) mobilization store, and (3) main presynaptic store. *Miniature endplate potentials (MEPP)* are small nonpropagating local depolarizations of the postsynaptic membrane caused by the random spontaneous release of single quanta of Ach. *Endplate potentials (EPP)* are graded local potentials of the endplate region caused by a nerve stimulus that results in a calcium-mediated release of approximately 100 to 200 quanta of Ach from the immediate store (Fig. 17-1). They can only be recorded if the ensuing muscle action potential is blocked. The calcium that enters the motor nerve terminal diffuses out in 100 to 200 msec. Repetitive stimulation rates in excess of 5 Hz (interstimulus interval of less than 200 msec) will therefore result in an accumulation of calcium and facilitate release of Ach, whereas slower rates will cause depletion of Ach. When the EPP reaches a critical threshold it generates a *muscle fiber action potential*, which results in a muscle contraction (Fig. 17-1). The EPP generated by a nerve impulse is normally always greater than the motor threshold ("safety factor") so that each impulse is followed by a muscle contraction (Fig. 17-1).

Slow repetitive stimulation results in a decrease in the number of quanta of Ach released with each impulse up to the fifth (Fig. 17-1) because the store of immediately available neurotransmitter quanta is depleted and the mobilization cannot keep pace with release. In disorders of the neuromuscular junction the safety factor is reduced so that the EPP may only reach threshold with the first few impulses in a train of stimuli and thus, the later impulses fail to be transmitted (Fig. 17-

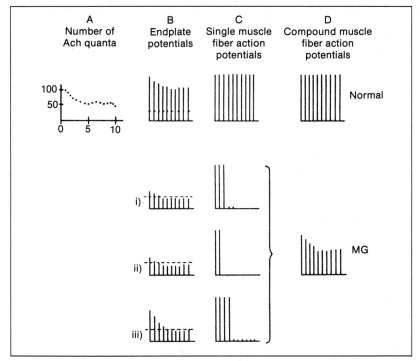

Figure 17-1. *Slow repetitive stimulation of a motor nerve showing the relationship between the release of acetylcholine (Ach) (A), the generation of endplate potentials (B), and the generation of single muscle fiber action potentials (C) in normal muscle (above) and in myasthenia gravis (MG) (below). Note that in MG the threshold (broken line) is not reached by the later stimuli in the train because of a reduced safety factor. D. Generation of compound muscle fiber action potentials in normal muscle (above) and a typical decrementing response in myasthenia gravis (below). (From D. Sanders. Electrophysiologic Study of Disorders of Neuromuscular Transmission. In M. J. Aminoff [Ed.],* Electrodiagnosis in Clinical Neurology *[2nd ed.]. New York: Churchill Livingstone, 1986. Used by permission.)*

1). This manifests as a decrement of the *compound muscle action potential (CMAP)*, which is a summation of the electrical activity of muscle fibers (Fig. 17-1). *Postactivation facilitation* refers to an increased release of Ach causing an increase in the EPP amplitude with rapid stimulation or following a short period of sustained voluntary contraction. Facilitation is due to the accumulation of calcium in the terminals and lasts for up to two minutes after the stimulation or contraction. The post activation facilitation is followed for up to 5 to 15 minutes by a decrease in Ach quanta release and reduced EPP amplitude (postactivation exhaustion) because of poorly understood metabolic changes. Normal muscles do not show any CMAP decrement, postactivation facilitation, or exhaustion because the EPP amplitude is always greater than the motor threshold.

Applications

Repetitive stimulation is a simple and useful test that can provide objective evidence of any dysfunction in neuromuscular transmission. Neuromuscular junction disorders may be presynaptic, like the Lambert-Eaton myasthenic syndrome (LEMS) [13] and botulism [2], or postsynaptic, like myasthenia gravis [10,12]. Abnormalities on repetitive stimulation in myasthenia gravis are seen in 50 to 95 percent [7,10,11,12] of cases, whereas the test is positive in all patients with the myasthenic syndrome.

Procedure

Site Selection (Table 17-1)

Any mixed or motor nerve can be tested provided adequate immobilization of stimulating and recording electrodes can be achieved. The electrodes are applied as for motor nerve conduction studies. Immobilization should include the muscle and the joints it moves so that contractions of the muscle are isometric (Fig. 17-2).

In myasthenia gravis the diagnostic yield is higher and the decrement more prominent at proximal sites [8,10]. However, a distal site should be tried first because proximal sites are more difficult to immobilize, have an unstable stimulus, and are more painful. In myasthenic syndrome all muscles are equally affected, so a distal site like the ulnar with hypothenar recording should be chosen. Muscle involvement with botulism can be more selective and, therefore, multiple test sites may need to be used.

Technical Considerations to Prevent Artifactual Changes

1. The stimulating and recording electrodes must be adequately immobilized (Fig. 17-2).
2. Stimuli must be supramaximal (at least 25% above maximal).
3. Stimulation rates of 2 to 3 Hz are optimal [3] for demonstrating dec-

Table 17-1. *Site Selection for Repetitive Stimulation*

Nerve	Stimulation	Recording	Excercise
Ulnar	Wrist	Hypothenar	Abduct little finger against strap
Median	Wrist	Thenar	Abduct thumb against strap
MC[a]	Axilla	Biceps	Flex supinated restrained forearm
Axillary	Erbs	Deltoid	Abduct restrained arm
Facial	Behind ear	Nasalis	Wrinkle nose
Accessory	SM[b]	Trapezius	Seated, holds chair, shrugs shoulder
Peroneal	Knee	Anterior tibial	Dorsiflex restrained foot

[a] Musculocutaneous.
[b] Posterior border of middle of sternomastoid.

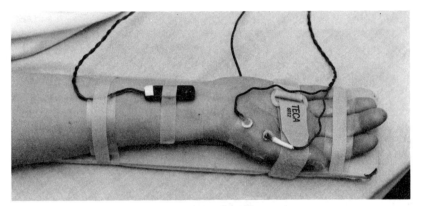

Figure 17-2. *Electrode placement for repetitive stimulation of the median nerve. The bipolar stimulating electrode is easier to immobilize.*

rement because they are fast enough to cause depletion of Ach at the motor terminal and yet slow enough to prevent calcium from accumulating.
4. Stimuli should be at least 6 to 9 per train to optimally demonstrate the different pattern of abnormalities.
5. The muscle should be rested at least 30 seconds between trials.
6. The skin temperature should be 33° to 35°C. Decrement with repetitive stimulation may improve in the myasthenic muscle at lower temperatures due to improved neuromuscular transmission [1].
7. Anticholinesterase medications can mask a decrement and may need to be stopped for a few hours prior to the study.

Test Procedure
The following sequence avoids unnecessary stimulations and is adequate for assessing the neuromuscular junction in a weak muscle.

1. Test the muscle at rest with a train of 6 to 9 supramaximal stimuli at 2 to 3 Hz frequency (optimal rate for demonstrating decrement). If a decrement is seen it should be reproducible after 30 seconds of rest.
2. Voluntary activation consists of a 10 to 20 second sustained voluntary isometric contraction (equivalent to firing rates of 20 to 40 Hz). The longer duration of voluntary contraction should be used if the muscle weakness is mild.
3. Repeat the train of 6 to 9 supramaximal stimuli at 2 to 3 Hz frequency immediately after activation (for postactivation facilitation). Postactivation increment is best seen within 10 seconds of the contraction after which it declines rapidly [3].
4. Test the muscle for postactivation exhaustion at 2 minutes and 4 minutes after the voluntary isometric contraction.

5. Alternate activation methods
    a. Voluntary contraction for 1 minute broken into three 20-second periods with 2 to 3 seconds in between is better for demonstrating postactivation exhaustion in patients with mild myasthenia gravis.
    b. Rapid stimulation rates of 20 to 50 Hz for 2 to 10 seconds may be used for activation in patients who cannot provide a sustained voluntary isometric contraction. Rapid rates cause pain with voluntary withdrawl and movement and are rarely needed.

Figure 17-3. *Repetitive stimulation showing a normal response* (top) *and a typical decrementing response in myasthenia gravis* (middle). *Pseudofacilitation* (bottom) *is recognized by a decrease in duration with increasing amplitude. (From D. Sanders. Electrophysiologic study of disorders of neuromuscular transmission. In M. J. Aminoff [Ed.],* Electrodiagnosis in Clinical Neurology *[2nd ed.]. New York: Churchill Livingstone, 1986. Used by permission.)*

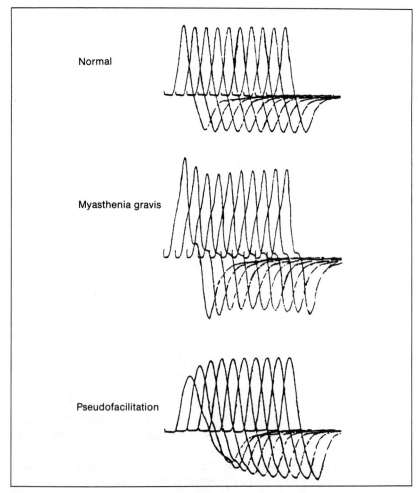

Normal

Myasthenia gravis

Pseudofacilitation

Table 17-2. *Decrement/Increment with Repetitive Stimulation*

Parameter	Normal	Myasthenia gravis	Myasthenic syndrome
Size of CMAP	Normal	Normal	Small
Decrement	None	>10%	>10%
Postactivation increment	<50%	<100%	>100%
Postactivation decrement repair	−	+	+
Postactivation exhaustion	−	+	+

Decrement
The decrement is calculated as the *maximum change in amplitude* expressed as a percentage of the first response [9]. Since the fourth or fifth response is usually the smallest in a series of decrementing responses, it is calculated between the first response and the fourth or fifth response. A true decrement demonstrates a smooth progression with the maximal change in CMAP amplitude between the first and second responses and a progressive decline to about the fourth or fifth response, followed by a transient increase in amplitude and then a long slow decrement (see Fig. 17-3). The decrement should be reproducible after a rest of 30 seconds and, ideally, should be demonstrated in at least two muscles. Abrupt or irregular changes in amplitude or waveform are frequently artifactual. Normal muscles show no decrement, but as a conservative approach, a decrement of greater than 8 to 10 percent (Table 17-2) is considered significant [10]. Decrement is characteristic of myasthenia gravis (Figs. 17-3, 17-4) but its absence does not exclude the diagnosis. Decrement is also seen in presynaptic disorders such as myasthenic syndrome, reinnervation, and some primary muscle diseases (see Chapter 20).

Postactivation Facilitation
Postactivation facilitation refers to the increment in the initial CMAP immediately after the 10-second activation (voluntary isometric contraction or tetanic nerve stimulation) and to the "repair of decrement" (decrease in rate of decrement). The increment is calculated as the maximal increase in amplitude as a percentage of the original response [9]. The maximal change is usually between the original response and the first postactivation response. Marked postactivation increment of 2 to 20 times the original response (Table 17-2) is characteristic of presynaptic disorders such as Lambert-Eaton myasthenic syndrome (LEMS). A low amplitude of the original CMAP (often 10 percent of normal mean amplitude) is consistently seen in LEMS (Fig. 17-4) and is almost a

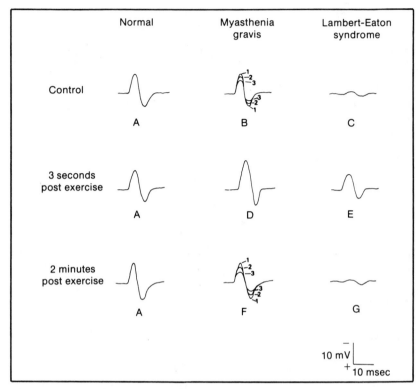

Figure 17-4. Normal response (A)—*no change.* **Myasthenia gravis**—*decrement at rest* (B); *postactivation increment* (D); *and postactivation exhaustion with a larger decrement than before exercise* (F). **Lambert-Eaton myasthenic syndrome**—*low amplitude baseline CMAP with a decremental response (decrement is not seen here due to low amplification)* (C); *marked postexercise increase in amplitude of CMAP combined with repair of decrement* (E) *and postactivation exhaustion with reduction of amplitude of CMAP to below baseline.*

diagnostic prerequisite [4]. Facilitation can also be identified by demonstrating an incrementing response with rapid repetitive stimulation (Fig. 17-5).

Normal muscles can show a postactivation increment of up to 40 to 50 percent [9,10,11]. This is referred to as *pseudofacilitation* because it results from an increased synchrony of conduction in muscle fibers rather than recruitment of additional muscle fibers. It is easily recognized because the increased amplitude is accompanied by a decrease in duration of the response and, therefore, the area remains unchanged (Fig. 17-3).

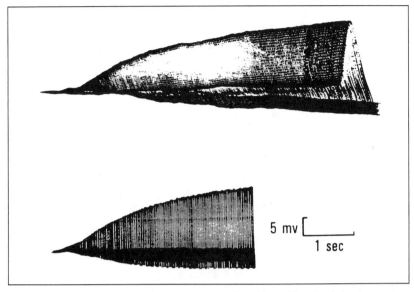

Figure 17-5. Incrementing ulnar motor response with rapid repetitive stimulation in a patient with Lambert-Eaton myasthenic syndrome. (From C. Jablecki. Lambert-Eaton myasthenic syndrome. Muscle Nerve 7:253, 1984. Used by permission.)

Postactivation Exhaustion

Postactivation exhaustion occurs 2 to 4 minutes after activation. It refers to the decrease in amplitude of the first CMAP below the original response and the increase in the amount of decrement above that which occurs in the pre-activation train of stimuli. It is seen in both pre- and postsynaptic neuromuscular junction disorders (Fig. 17-4).

References

1. Borenstein, S., and Desmedt, J. G.   New Diagnostic Procedures in Myasthenia Gravis. In J. E. Desmedt (Ed), *New Developments in EMG and Clinical Neurophysiology*. Vol. 1. Basel: Karger, 1973.
2. Cherington, M.   Botulism: Ten-year experience. *Arch. Neurol.* 30:432, 1974.
3. Desmedt, J. E., (Ed.).   The Neuromuscular Disorder in Myasthenia Gravis. *New Developments in EMG and Clinical Neurophysiology*. Vol. 1. Basel: Karger, 1973.
4. Henriksson, K. G., Nilson, O., Rosen, I., et al.   Clinical, neurophysiological, and morphological findings in Eaton-Lambert syndrome. *Acta. Neurol. Scand.*, 56:117, 1970.

5. Hubbard, J. I.   Microphysiology of vertebrate neuromuscular transmission. *Physiologic Reviews* 53(3):674, 1973.
6. Jablecki, C.   Lambert-Eaton myasthenic syndrome. *Muscle Nerve.* 7:250, 1984.
7. Kelly, J. J., Jr., Daube, J. R., Lennon, V. A., et al.   The laboratory diagnosis of mild myasthenia gravis. *Ann. Neurol.* 12:238, 1982.
8. Krarup, C.   Electrical and Mechanical responses in the platysma and in the adductor pollicis muscle. *J. Neurol. Neurosurg. Psychiatry.* 40:241, 1977.
9. Lange, D. J.   The Eaton-Lambert syndrome: Current concepts of pathogenesis and treatment. *Neurology and Neurosurgery Update Series,* 4(26):1, 1983.
10. Ozdemir, C., and Young, R. R.   The results to be expected from electrical testing in the diagnosis of myasthenia gravis. *Ann. N. Y. Acad. Sci.* 274:203, 1976.
11. Sanders, D. M.   Electrophysiologic Study of Disorders of Neuromuscular Transmission. In M. J. Aminoff, (Ed.), *Electrodiagnosis in Clinical Neurology.* New York: Churchill Livingstone, 1986.
12. Stalberg, E.   Clinical electrophysiology of myasthenia gravis. *J. Neurol. Neurosurg. Psychiatry.* 43:622, 1980.
13. Swift, T. R.   Disorders of neuromuscular transmission other than myasthenia gravis. *Muscle Nerve.* 334, 1981.

The EMG Examination 18

Because there are more than 430 skeletal muscles in the human body and patchy involvement of muscles may exist in some neuromuscular diseases, it is impossible to completely standardize the needle examination. The clinical examination forms the basis for planning an appropriate needle examination in an individual patient, and the extent of the testing often depends upon what is found in the initially tested muscles. A knowledge of the root and peripheral nerve innervation (see Appendixes V, VI) and surface anatomy of commonly studied muscles (see Appendix VII) is essential in planning an appropriate examination and in interpreting the results. The recommended EMG machine settings are given in Appendix I.

Anatomy and Physiology

The *motor unit* is the smallest functional unit of the motor system and consists of a motor neuron, its axon, and all the muscle fibers innervated by the axon. *Innervation ratio* refers to the ratio of muscle fibers to the innervating axons and is an estimate of the size of the motor unit. Muscles subserving fine movements tend to have smaller innervation ratios than those subserving coarse movement. Large motor neurons innervate a greater number of muscle fibers and have larger innervation ratios. The average motor unit territory determined by a multilead electrode is 5 to 10 mm [5] with the muscle fibers widely scattered over this area. The territory of a motor unit allows space for fibers of 10 to 30 overlapping motor units [3]. Recruitment of motor units follows the "size principle" [13,14], which states that voluntary activation of smaller motor neurons occurs before larger motor neurons. Muscle fibers are essentially of two types, and those belonging to a given motor unit are always of the same type. *Type I fibers* belong to the smaller, initially recruited motor units and are the ones primarily assessed with electromyography [30]. They are rich in oxidative enzymes and are resistant to fatigue. *Type II fibers* belong to larger motor neurons that are recruited with greater effort and are low in oxidative enzymes and fatigue easily.

Recording Electrodes

Two main types of needle electrodes (Fig. 18-1) are used in electromyographic recording, the outer diameter of both being less than 1 mm. *123*

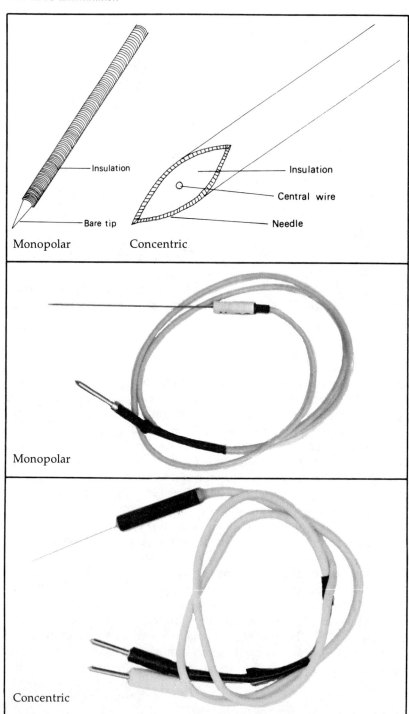

Figure 18-1. *Monopolar and bipolar electrodes.*

The Concentric (Coaxial) Electrode (Fig. 18-1)
The concentric electrode consists of an outer stainless steel cannula through which runs a single wire that is exposed at its tip. The inner wire serves as the recording electrode, the outer cannula serves as the reference electrode, and the potential difference between the two is recorded. A separate ground is used.

Monopolar Needle Electrode (Fig. 18-1)
The monopolar needle electrode is a solid steel electrode covered with insulation (usually Teflon) except at its tip. This electrode serves as the G_1 or active recording electrode; a second reference electrode, G_2 (either needle or surface), must be placed nearby (Fig. 18-2). The potential difference between the active and reference electrodes is measured in EMG. A separate ground is also used. The variabilities in the position of the reference electrode and changes in the recording area on the needle tip (from Teflon retraction) can affect the motor unit potential characteristics with monopolar recordings. Table 18-1 lists differences between the two types of electrodes.

During a needle examination, insertional activity, spontaneous activity, and exertional activity are routinely assessed.

Insertional Activity
As the needle electrode enters or is moved within a muscle, fibers are mechanically stimulated, cut, and injured. These alterations of the mus-

Figure 18-2. Monopolar electrode placement.

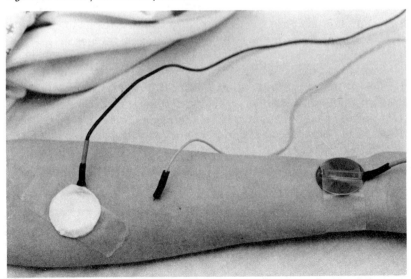

Table 18-1. *Needle Electrode Characteristics*

Parameter	Monopolar	Concentric
Motor unit potential		
Recording area	Larger	Smaller
Amplitude	Larger	Smaller
Total duration	Similar	Similar
Major spike duration	Longer	Shorter
Patient discomfort	Less painful	More painful
Expense	Inexpensive	Expensive

cle cells give rise to bursts of potentials. A single burst should not last more than 300 to 500 msec after the movement of the needle ceases (Fig. 18-3). Prolonged insertional activity may be an early indication of denervation, but can also be seen in inflammatory myopathies and myotonic disorders. Reduced insertional activity is seen with fibrosis, with fatty replacement of normal muscle, or during attacks of familial periodic paralysis.

Spontaneous Activity

Spontaneous activity occurring after insertional activity has ceased is abnormal with some exceptions.

Normal Spontaneous Activity

Normal muscle at rest is electrically silent except in the endplate region (the zone of innervation located in the middle of the muscle) where at least two types of endplate activity (Fig. 18-4) may be identified separately or simultaneously [12]. Electrode insertion in the endplate region is accompanied by pain that is relieved by moving the needle.

ENDPLATE NOISE. Endplate noise is low amplitude undulating activity (Fig. 18-4) that sounds like a seashell held to the ear. Endplate noise represents nonpropagated endplate depolarizations (miniature endplate potentials) caused by the random spontaneous release of single quanta (vesicles) of acetylcholine from the motor nerve terminals.

ENDPLATE SPIKES. Endplate spikes are nonpropagated single muscle fiber

Figure 18-3. *Normal insertional activity (A = point of needle insertion or movement).*

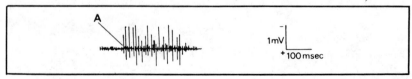

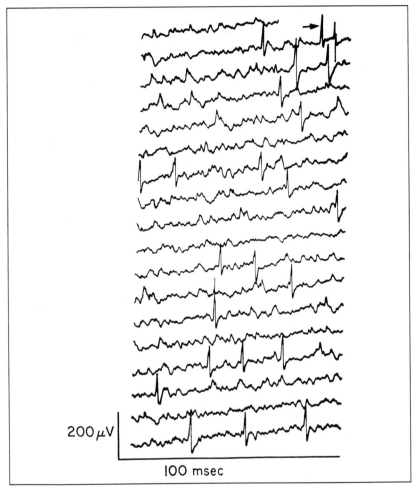

Figure 18-4. *Normal endplate activity: low amplitude undulating endplate noise and endplate spikes* (arrow). *Note the initial negativity (upward deflection) of the endplate spikes.*

discharges caused by excitation in the intramuscular nerves. Table 18-2 lists the characteristics which help in the recognition of this physiologic endplate activity. It is important to differentiate the normal endplate spikes, which are always initially negative (upward) and often accompanied by the hissing endplate noise, from fibrillations that have similar amplitude and duration but are initially positive (downward).

Abnormal Spontaneous Activity

Fibrillations and Positive Sharp Waves. *Fibrillations* are spontaneously firing action potentials originating from denervated single muscle fibers

Table 18-2. *Normal Spontaneous Activity*

Parameter	Endplate noise	Endplate spikes
Amplitude	10–50 μV	100–200 μV
Duration	1–2 msec	3–5 msec
Frequency	20–40 Hz	5–50 Hz
Firing interval	Irregular	Irregular
Sound	Hissing	Crackling
Configuration	Monophasic (negative)	Diphasic (initial negative)

recorded extracellularly (see Fig. 18-5). When recorded outside the end-plate region they have an initial positive phase (Table 18-3) and a total of two or three phases.

Positive sharp waves are potentials recorded with the needle electrode very near a denervated discharging muscle fiber and usually accompany

Figure 18-5. *Fibrillations* (A) *and positive sharp waves* (B). *The faster sweep* (above) *demonstrates the duration of the potentials more clearly.*

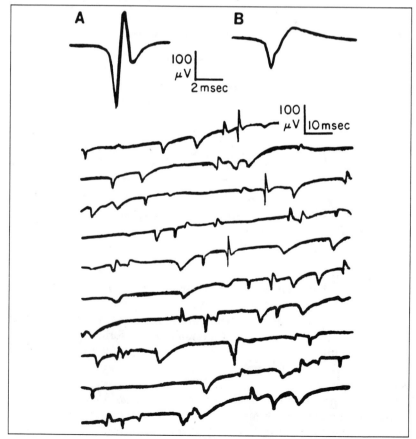

Table 18-3. *Denervation Activity*

Parameters	Fibrillations	Positive sharp waves
Amplitude (peak to peak)	20–300 μV (<1 mV)	20–300 μV (<1 mV)
Duration	1–5 msec	10–30 msec (<100 msec)
Frequency	1–50 Hz	1–50 Hz
Firing interval	Usually regular	Usually regular
Sound	Crisp clicks	Dull popping
Configuration	Bi- or triphasic (initial positive, then sharp negative)	Biphasic (initial sharp positive then long negative wave)

fibrillation potentials. They are diphasic potentials (Table 18-3) with an abrupt initial positive deflection followed by a slow negative decay (Fig. 18-5). On occasion, movement of the EMG needle will demonstrate a transition from fibrillations to positive waves in a single fiber.

Fibrillations and positive sharp waves can be graded either by the number of sites within the muscle in which they are seen or as follows [16].

1+ Transient following needle movement
2+ Occasional, at rest in more than two sites
3+ Present, at rest in most sites
4+ Abundant, almost filling the screen at all sites

Fibrillations and positive sharp waves have the same clinical significance and should be seen in at least two sites to be considered abnormal. They are most often seen in neurogenic lesions affecting the anterior horn cells, roots, plexus, or peripheral nerves. They take 2 to 5 weeks to appear following nerve injury depending on the distance between the injury site to the recording muscle. Fibrillations and positive sharp waves may also be seen in primary muscle diseases, particularly inflammatory myopathies and muscular dystrophies. Muscle necrosis with intramuscular denervation of muscle fibers may be partly responsible for their presence in muscle diseases [10]. Neuromuscular junction disorders like botulism are occasionally associated with fibrillations and positive sharp waves. Positive waves and fibrillation potentials have been reported in patients with upper motor neuron lesions [15], but this observation is probably due to a superimposed lower motor neuron lesion such as a traction or compression neuropathy [8].

FASCICULATIONS. A fasciculation is the nonvolitional, random contraction of a group of muscle fibers representing a whole or part of a motor unit. A fasciculation may cause visible movements of the skin and mucous membrane (tongue) or of a small joint. A fasciculation potential is the electrical potential associated with visible fasciculation (Fig. 18-6). Fas-

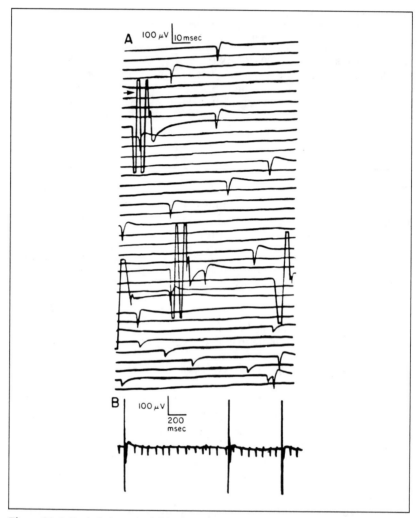

Figure 18-6. *Fasciculation potential* (arrow) *with accompanying positive sharp waves recorded in raster mode* (A) *and continuous mode* (B). *Note the irregular firing of the fasciculation potentials.*

ciculations are most commonly, but not exclusively, found in neurogenic lesions. They are seen with neurogenic lesions at any site from the cell body to the motor nerve terminal but are most frequent in patients with proximal neuropathies such as motor neuron disease and irritative lesions of spinal nerve roots. Fasciculations may occur in patients with thyrotoxicosis and are also seen in normal individuals, especially in the calf muscles and in the small muscles of the hand and feet. "Benign" fasciculations cannot reliably be distinguished from "malignant" fasciculation potentials resulting from specific disease. Benign fasciculations generally have a faster frequency (average 0.8 Hz) and simpler waveform compared with an average interval of 3.5 seconds in motor neuron disease [27]. A summary of the characteristics of the fasciculations is given below:

Duration	Variable (usually 3 to 15 msec)
Amplitude	Variable (usually 300 μV to 3 mV)
Configuration	Triphasic to polyphasic
Repetition frequency	0.1 to 10 per second
Firing interval	Irregular
Sound	Dull pop

COMPLEX REPETITIVE DISCHARGES. Complex repetitive discharges (CRDs) are action potentials of a group of muscle fibers firing in near synchrony (Fig. 18-7). Single fiber recordings show up to 10 single fiber potentials within each complex [28]. They were previously referred to as bizarre high-frequency discharges or pseudomyotonia. These trains of potentials can have a variable frequency (5 to 100 Hz), amplitude (100 μV to 1 mV), and duration. The waveform may be simple or complex (Fig. 18-7) [1]. They usually have an abrupt onset and cessation and their amplitude, frequency, and waveform remain constant within any single train, although a sudden change in shape can occur (Fig. 18-7B). They lack the characteristic waxing and waning quality of myotonic discharges (Fig. 18-8) from which they need to be differentiated. CRDs are nonspecific and may be seen in a wide variety of neurogenic and myopathic disorders. Patients with myxedema and metabolic diseases such as acid maltase deficiency may show prominent CRDs.

MYOTONIC DISCHARGES. Myotonic discharges (Fig. 18-8) are single-fiber action potentials whose waveform is that of positive sharp waves or

Figure 18-7. Complex repetitive discharges with a firing frequency of 30 Hz (A), 50–80 Hz (B), and 70 Hz (C). The amplitude, waveform and frequency are constant but may abruptly change within the same discharge (B). The waveform may be simple (B) or complex (C).

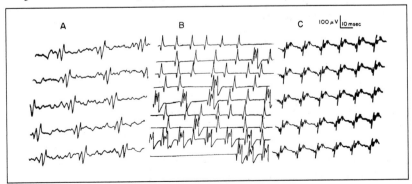

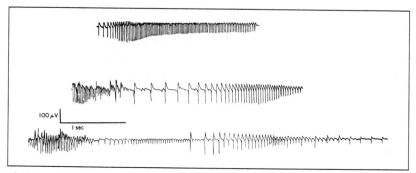

Figure 18-8. *Myotonic discharges. Note the simple configuration and the marked variation in amplitude and frequency within the discharge.*

fibrillations. Myotonic discharges wax and wane in frequency (20 to 150 Hz) and amplitude (10 μV to 1 mV), giving a characteristic "dive-bomber" sound over the loudspeaker. They are triggered by needle movement, percussion of the muscle, or voluntary contraction. Myotonic discharges are seen in myotonic dystrophy, myotonia congenita, paramyotonia congenita, and hyperkalemic periodic paralysis [16].

MYOKYMIA. Myokymia is a spontaneous slow contraction of small bands of muscle fibers that gives a rippling appearance to the overlying skin [29]. Myokymia represents a sustained contraction which should be distinguished from the single twitch of a fasciculation. Myokymic discharges are groups of motor unit action potentials that fire repetitively and may be associated with clinical myokymia. Myokymic discharges have two electromyographic patterns [1]: (1) involuntary, spontaneously occurring bursts of several motor unit potentials discharging rhythmically at frequencies of 1 to 5 Hz (Fig. 18-9A) and (2) single or paired motor units firing repetitively for a short period (up to a few seconds) at a uniform rate (2 to 60 Hz) followed by a short period of silence (up to a few seconds) (Fig. 18-9B). The latter should be differentiated from doublets or multiplets, which are under voluntary control.

These grouped discharges occur independently in different areas of the muscle. The motor unit potentials within a given group are identical and fire at rapid frequencies (Fig. 18-9A). However, the pattern of firing varies both in the same muscle and in different muscles when present in multiple locations [2]. The discharges are seen in neurogenic lesions affecting any portion of the motor neuron from the cell body to the distal nerve terminals. Clinical myokymia is often seen in facial muscles and less commonly in limb muscles.

Facial myokymia has been reported with multiple sclerosis (lasting

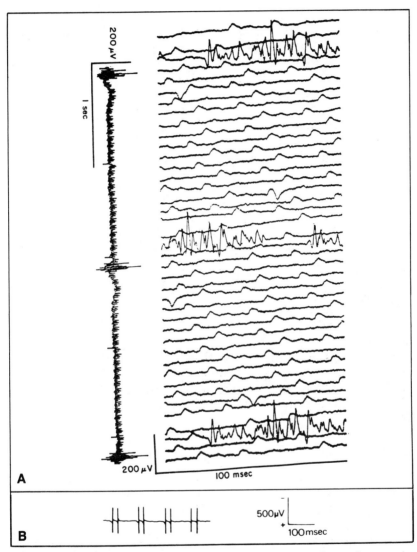

200 μV

1 sec

200 μV   100 msec

A

500μV
100 msec

B

Figure 18-9. *Myokymic discharges. A. Involuntary spontaneous bursts of grouped motor unit potentials discharging rhythmically. B. Single or paired motor units fire repetitively followed by a short period of silence.*

from weeks to years), brainstem neoplasms (generally persistent), and in patients with inflammatory polyradiculopathy [9,23].

Limb myokymia is most often seen in patients with radiation-induced plexopathy and less commonly in radiation-induced radiculopathy or radiation myelopathy [2]. Patients without radiation are a heterogeneous group with neurogenic lesions, the most common of which are acute and chronic radiculoneuropathies and chronic nerve entrapments.

NEUROMYOTONIC DISCHARGES. Neuromyotonia, or continuous muscle fiber activity (Isaac's syndrome), is a clinical syndrome with continuous muscle rippling and stiffness [1]. Neuromyotonic discharges are high-frequency (150 to 300 Hz) bursts of decrementing discharges of motor unit potentials that originate in motor axons (Fig. 18-10). They start and end abruptly and typically result in characteristically high-pitched musical pings over the loudspeaker [16]. The discharges may be spontaneous or initiated by needle movement, voluntary contraction, or percussion of the nerve. Motor and sensory nerve conductions may be at the lower normal limits. This condition is improved by the administration of phenytoin or carbamazepine. Neuromyotonic discharges can also be seen with chronic neuropathies and in spinal muscular atrophy [18].

CRAMP. A cramp is a transient involuntary painful muscular contraction that may result from unaccustomed exertion, sodium depletion, uremia, myxedema, hypocalcemia, alkalosis, or drugs but whose origin is most often unexplained. The EMG reflects the full interference pattern of maximal effort or may demonstrate only a few rapidly firing motor units in the vicinity of the needle.

Stiff-Man Syndrome. The stiff-man syndrome [20] is a rare sporadic disorder in which symmetrical continuous stiffness with uncontrollable and painful spasms of the muscles develops. The EMG reveals continuous, normal-appearing motor unit activity that persists in the absence of effort but disappears with sleep. These persistent tonic contractions represent hyperactivity of the gamma system and can be relieved by diazepam.

CONTRACTURE. A contracture must be differentiated from a cramp. Contracture refes to an electrically silent shortening of the muscles induced by exertion. It can be seen in McArdle's disease (phosphorylase deficiency) and phosphofructokinase deficiency [29].

Figure 18-10. *Neuromyotonic discharge. Note the high frequency and decrementing nature of the discharge. (From W. Litchy. Needle examination in electromyography.* Course A: Basic Nerve Conduction and Electromyography. *American Association of Electromyography and Electrodiagnosis, Boston, MA, 1986. Used by permission.)*

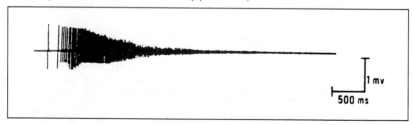

Tremor Studies. In patients with tremors, the pattern of EMG activity in antagonistic muscles (e.g., forearm flexors and extensors) can be recorded on two separate channels using either surface disc electrodes or needle electrodes. Low-frequency components of the EMG are restricted by the use of a 500-Hz low-frequency filter. A sweep velocity of 200 msec/cm is optimal. The initial machine settings for tremor studies are given in Appendix I. The frequency of tremor and the pattern of contraction in antagonistic muscle is useful in the differentiation of different types of tremors [26] as follows.

1. *Physiologic tremor:* frequency 8 to 12 Hz; synchronous in antagonistic muscles; best seen with arms outstretched (postural) [26].
2. *Essential tremor:* frequency 5 to 8 Hz; synchronous in antagonistic muscles (Fig. 18-11); best seen with arms outstretched (postural). Neuropathic tremor in patients with peripheral neuropathies may have similar characteristics [26].
3. *Parkinsonian tremor:* frequency 3 to 7 Hz; alternates between antagonistic muscles (Fig. 18-11); best seen at rest and at least briefly suppressed during voluntary activity [26]. Extrapyramidal disorders besides Parkinson's disease may have a tremor with similar characteristics.
4. *Rubral (cerebellar outflow) tremor:* frequency 2.5 to 4.0 Hz; alternates in antagonistic muscles; best seen with arms outstretched (postural)

Figure 18-11. *Tremor recording over forearm flexors and extensors. (A) Parkinsonian tremor—4 Hz alternating in antagonistic muscles; and (B) essential tremor—8 Hz synchronous in antagonistic muscles.*

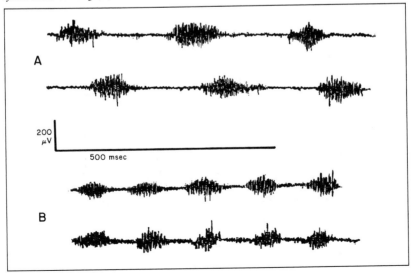

and more prominent in proximal muscles [24]. Cerebellar intention tremor without postural tremor is better appreciated clinically than with EMG.

Exertional Activity

A motor unit action potential (MUAP) is seen when the muscle is voluntarily activated and represents the summated electrical activity of the muscle fibers innervated by a single motor unit that are within the recording range of the recording electrode. The electrical activity approaching, reaching, and leaving the recording extracellular needle electrode within a volume conductor generates a MUAP waveform that is usually triphasic (positive-negative-positive) in configuration (Fig. 18-12). MUAPs are characterized by their appearance and firing pattern. With careful electrode placement and a cooperative patient who is able to control a minimal effort, a single MUAP can be displayed on the oscilloscope (Fig. 18-13). It is useful to "freeze" this unit using a trigger and delay line and store or photograph it for more careful study when first learning to appreciate the enormous range of normal variations of the MUAP.

For quantitative measurements, 2 to 3 initially activated units are taken from each site. Each unit should be clearly identified in its entirety at least twice to prevent false measurement of overlapped potentials (Fig. 18-13). Several sites can be examined with a single needle puncture

Figure 18-12. Measured parameters of a motor unit action potential (MUAP).

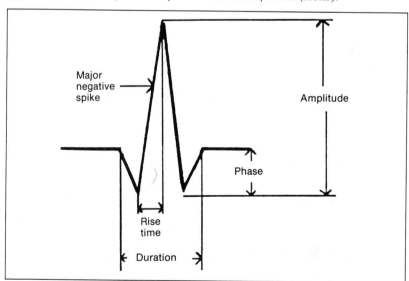

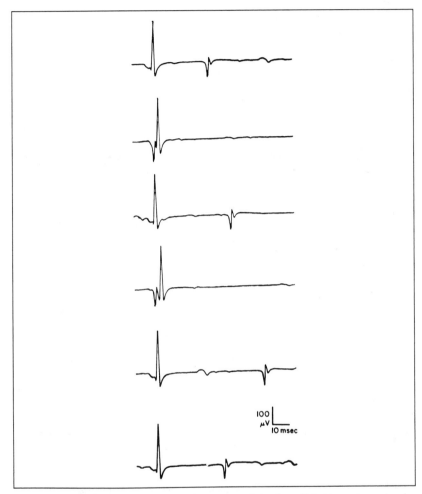

Figure 18-13. *Normal motor units. The first motor unit is ''frozen'' in place using a signal trigger and delay line. For quantitative measurements the potential should be seen in its entirety at least twice to prevent measuring overlapped potentials like the 2nd and 4th triggered potential in this recording.*

by advancing or withdrawing the needle in small steps and changing the direction of the needle two or three times. Amplitude, duration, and incidence of polyphasic potentials are measured for 20 or more MUAPs recorded with mild contraction. A normal mean duration of at least 20 motor units should be within 20 percent of the mean for age (Table 18-4). Quantitative studies are more objective but are time-consuming, although computer measurements on the newer machines have simplified the task. The essential characteristics of the MUAP are as follows.

Table 18-4. *Mean Duration of Motor Unit Potentials*

Age (yr)	Frontalis	Biceps brachii	Triceps brachii	Extensor digitorum communis	Interosseous dorsalis I	Vastus medialis	Tibialis anterior	Gastrocnemius
0	4.1	7.7	9.0	7.1	7.7	7.9	9.5	7.2
3	4.4	8.2	9.6	7.6	8.2	8.4	10.1	7.7
5	4.5	8.5	9.9	7.8	8.5	8.7	10.5	8.0
8	4.7	8.9	10.3	8.2	8.9	9.1	11.0	8.4
10	4.8	9.1	10.6	8.4	9.1	9.3	11.2	8.6
13	5.0	9.4	11.0	8.7	9.4	9.6	11.6	8.8
15	5.1	9.6	11.2	8.8	9.6	9.8	11.7	8.9
18	5.2	9.8	11.4	9.0	9.8	10.0	12.1	9.2
20	5.3	10.0	11.6	9.2	10.0	10.2	12.3	9.4
25	5.3	10.3	11.9	9.5	10.3	10.5	12.7	9.7
30	5.4	10.6	12.0	9.8	10.6	10.8	13.1	10.0
35	5.4	10.9	12.1	10.0	10.9	11.1	13.4	10.2
40	5.5	11.1	12.2	10.2	11.1	11.3	13.6	10.4
45	5.5	11.2	12.3	10.3	11.2	11.4	13.8	10.5
50	5.6	11.4	12.4	10.5	11.4	11.6	14.0	10.7
55	5.6	11.6	12.5	10.7	11.6	11.8	14.3	10.9
60	5.7	11.9	12.6	11.0	11.9	12.1	14.7	11.2
65	5.7	12.2	12.7	11.2	12.2	12.4	15.0	11.5
70	5.8	12.4	12.8	11.4	12.4	12.6	15.3	11.7
75	5.8	12.6	12.8	11.6	12.6	12.8	15.5	11.8
80	5.9	12.8	12.8	11.8	12.8	13.0	15.7	12.0

Source: Values from Rigshospitalet Laboratory of Clinical Neurophysiology. *Electromyography: Sensory and Motor Conduction. Findings in Normal Subjects.* Copenhagen: Rigshopspitalet, 1975.

Amplitude	Variable (up to 3 mV)
Duration	Variable (<15 msec)
Frequency	Depends on degree of effort (up to 50 per second)
Configuration	2 to 3 phases; 5 to 12% polyphasic (more than 4 phases is considered polyphasic)
Firing pattern	Semirhythmic
Sound	Sharp and crisp (when rise time is <500 μsec)

The *rise time* is measured from the initial positive to the subsequent negative peak (see Fig. 18-12) and is a good indicator of the distance between the EMG needle tip and the muscle fibers generating the major spike potential of the motor unit being studied. The rise time should be less than 500 μsec for the MUAP to be acceptable for measurement [16]. As the appropriate fibers are approached, the rise time becomes shorter and the MUAP sound over the loudspeaker becomes sharp and crisp.

The *amplitude* of the major spike is primarily determined by the muscle fibers located near the tip of the recording needle electrode and is the most variable characteristic. The amplitude of single muscle fiber potentials falls to less than 10 percent at a distance of 1 mm from where they are generated because the intervening tissue acts like a high-frequency filter [11]. The fiber density and distance between the recording electrode and active muscle fibers determine the MUAP amplitude.

The *duration* of a MUAP, measured from the initial deflection from the baseline to final return to the baseline (see Fig. 18-12), is an important indicator of the size of the motor unit territory. The muscle acts as a high-frequency (low-pass) filter, so only low-frequency components of muscle fiber potentials located more than 1 mm from the needle electrode are recorded and make up the initial and terminal phases of the MUAP [5].

A *phase* is defined as the portion of the wave between the departure from and return to the baseline (see Fig. 18-12) and is measured as the number of baseline crossings plus one [1]. Polyphasic potentials have more than four phases and do not normally exceed 12 percent of the fibers measured in any one muscle (Table 18-5), except in the deltoid where polyphasic potentials up to 25 percent are normal [3]. However, very polyphasic units may be abnormal even if just a few are seen. If the degree of polyphasia observed is mild, 20 or more single motor unit potentials must be examined in a single muscle to determine the overall percentage of polyphasic units in a given muscle. Polarity reversals without baseline crossings are called *turns*, and potentials with increased number of turns are called *serrated potentials*. Polyphasic and serrated potentials are a measure of reduced muscle fiber synchrony. A *satellite potential* (Fig. 18-14) is a small action potential which is separate from but time-locked to the main action potential. Satellite potentials are seen in neurogenic disorders with immature reinnervated units and in myopathies with muscle fiber regeneration.

Table 18-5. *Polyphasic Potentials
in Normal Human Muscles*

Muscle	Polyphasic potentials (%)
Biceps brachii	3.5
Biceps femoris	4.5
Gastrocnemius	0.5
Tibialis anterior	8.5
Facial muscles	5.5
Extensor digitorum brevis	12.0

Source: Adapted from F. Buchthal and P. Rosenfalck. Action potential parameters in different human muscles. *Acta Psychiatr. Neurol. Scand.* 30:125, 1955. Used by permission.

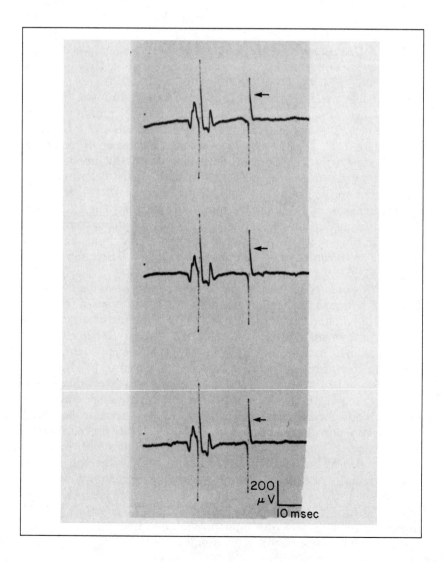

Physiologic Variables

MUSCLE-TO-MUSCLE VARIATION. The amplitude, duration, and number of phases of normal MUAPs vary greatly from muscle to muscle (Tables 18-6, 18-7). Amplitudes and durations are lower in the extraocular, facial, intercostal, and paraspinous muscles, which have lower innervation ratios, while they are higher in the limb muscles.

Table 18-6. *Durations of Motor Unit Action Potentials in Upper Extremity Muscles*

Age (yr)	Deltoid (msec)	Biceps brachii (msec)	Triceps brachii (msec)	Opponens pollicis (msec)	Abductor digiti quinti (msec)
0–4	7.9–10.1	6.4–8.2	7.2–9.3	7.1–9.1	8.3–10.6
5–9	8.0–10.8	6.5–8.8	7.3–9.9	7.2–9.8	8.4–11.4
10–14	8.1–11.2	6.6–9.1	7.5–10.3	7.3–10.1	8.5–11.7
15–19	8.6–12.2	7.0–9.9	7.9–11.2	7.8–11.0	9.0–12.8
20–29	9.5–13.2	7.7–10.7	8.7–12.1	8.5–11.9	9.9–13.8
30–39	11.1–14.9	9.0–12.1	10.2–13.7	10.0–13.4	11.6–15.6
40–49	11.8–15.7	9.6–12.8	10.9–14.5	10.7–14.2	12.4–16.5
50–59	12.8–16.7	10.4–13.6	11.8–15.4	11.5–15.1	13.4–17.5
60–69	13.3–17.3	10.8–14.1	12.2–15.9	12.0–15.7	13.9–18.2
70–79	13.7–17.7	11.1–14.4	12.5–16.3	12.3–16.0	14.3–18.6

Source: From F. Buchthal and P. Rosenfalck. Action potential parameters in different human muscles. *Acta Psychiatr. Neurol. Scand.* 30:125, 1955. Used by permission.

Table 18-7. *Durations of Motor Unit Action Potentials in Lower Extremity Muscles*

Age (yr)	Biceps femoris: quadriceps (msec)	Gastroc-nemius (msec)	Tibialis anterior (msec)	Peroneus longus (msec)	Extensor digitorum brevis (msec)
0–4	7.9–9.2	6.4–8.2	8.0–10.2	5.8–7.4	6.3–8.1
5–9	7.3–9.9	6.5–8.8	8.1–11.0	5.9–7.9	6.4–8.7
10–14	7.4–10.2	6.6–9.1	8.2–11.3	5.9–8.2	6.5–9.0
15–19	7.8–11.1	7.0–9.9	8.7–12.3	6.3–8.9	6.9–9.8
20–29	8.6–12.0	7.7–10.7	9.6–13.3	6.9–9.6	7.6–10.6
30–39	10.1–13.5	9.0–12.1	11.2–15.1	8.1–10.9	8.9–12.0
40–49	10.7–14.3	9.6–12.8	11.9–15.9	8.6–11.5	9.5–12.7
50–59	11.6–15.2	10.4–13.6	12.9–16.9	9.4–12.2	10.3–13.5
60–69	12.1–15.8	10.8–14.1	13.4–17.5	9.7–12.7	10.7–14.0
70–79	12.4–16.1	11.1–14.4	13.8–17.9	10.0–13.0	11.0–14.3

Source: From F. Buchthal and P. Rosenfalck. Action potential parameters in different human muscles. *Acta Psychiatr. Neurol. Scand.* 30:125, 1955. Used by permission.

Figure 18-14. *Satellite potential* (arrow) *is separate from but time-locked to the main potential.*

AGE. The average duration of the MUAPs increases from infancy to adult-hood (Table 18-8) due to growth in width of the muscle fibers over which the endplates are scattered [3,4,24]. In adults, there is a further increase from 20 to 70 years of age (see Table 18-5), probably from attrition of motor neurons and collateral sprouting.

TEMPERATURE. An increase of polyphasic potentials and in mean duration of MUAPs (10 percent per degree Celsius) is seen with a decrease in recording temperature [7].

SIZE PRINCIPLE. Increase in effort activates smaller units before larger ones [13].

Abnormalities in Motor Unit Action Potential Characteristics
MYOPATHIC DISORDERS. In patients with myopathy, the loss of distant fibers affects the initial and terminal phases of the MUAP with a short-ening of the mean duration of the recorded potential (Table 18-9). The

Table 18-8. *Variation of Duration, Amplitude, and Configuration of the MUAP (Concentric Electrode)*

Age	Mean duration ± standard error of the mean (msec)	Mean voltage (μV)	Polyphasic potentials in >4 phases (%)
Abductor Digiti Quinti			
3 months	5.8 ± 0.1	78 ± 12	0.6
16–23 years	9.4 ± 0.25	360 ± 20	3.3
26–40 years	9.1 ± 0.25	—	2.0
47–52 years	9.0 ± 0.3	—	4.7
61–80 years	10.1 ± 0.35	330 ± 50	4.4
Biceps Brachii			
3 months	7.7 ± 0.3	96 ± 7	6.0
16–23 years	10.3 ± 0.2	175 ± 20	2.8
26–40 years	10.9 ± 0.45	—	4.9
47–52 years	11.3 ± 0.35	—	4.9
61–80 years	12.7 ± 0.25	290 ± 40	3.8

Source: Adapted from G. Sacco, F. Buchthal, and P. Rosenfalck. Motor unit potentials at different ages. *Arch. Neurol.* 6:44, 1962. Copyright 1962, American Medical Association.

Table 18-9. *Typical MUAP Characteristics in Myopathic, Neuropathic, and Normal Muscle*

	Myopathy	Normal	Neuropathy
Duration	<5 msec	5–16 msec	>16 msec
Amplitude (mean)	<200 μV	200–400 μV	>400 μV
Configuration	Polyphasic	Triphasic	Polyphasic

mean amplitude may be reduced as a result of loss of fibers lying close to the electrode. There is an increase in polyphasic units because the spikes from the surviving muscle fibers are widely separated in time (Fig. 18-15). Satellite potentials can also be seen in myopathies and indicate regeneration from myotubes, which have a much slower conduction velocity [6].

Neuromuscular junction disorders such as myasthenia gravis, myasthenic syndrome, and botulism have functional loss of muscle fibers. They either have a normal EMG or have MUAP abnormalities similar to patients with myopathic disorders. In addition, patients with disorders of neuromuscular transmission may have variation in MUAP morphology (especially amplitude) during continuous activity. This variability of MUAPs is due to impaired activation or blocking of single muscle fibers and can also be seen in reinnervated units.

NEUROPATHIC DISORDERS. In neuropathic disorders, the reinnervation of denervated muscle fibers by collaterals from surviving motor neurons results in an increase in the average number of muscle fibers per motor unit. Therefore, a greater number of fibers in the same motor unit will be within the range of the EMG needle, and thus the mean duration and amplitude of the motor unit action potential is increased (Table 18-9). Amplitude is so variable in normal MUAPs that only extremes of amplitude can be considered abnormal. There is an increase in polyphasia (Fig. 18-15) due to asynchronous firing of muscle fiber potentials resulting from a greater anatomic scatter of individual endplates and slower conduction in immature collaterals. The polyphasia tends to be more prominent early in the course of reinnervation. Highly polyphasic, low-amplitude, long-duration motor units are observed during early stages of reinnervation after complete denervation of the muscle and have been termed nascent units [1].

Figure 18-15. Motor unit action potentials. A. Neuropathic—large, prolonged, polyphasic. B. Myopathic—small, short, polyphasic. C. Normal.

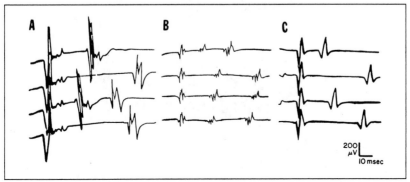

Firing Pattern

Tension in a voluntarily contracted muscle is initially due to an increased firing rate and subsequently due to an increased number of motor units. *Recruitment* refers to this successive activation of additional motor units with increased strength. The *onset frequency* is the lowest stable frequency that can be voluntarily maintained for a single motor unit (Fig. 18-16); for an average motor unit it is about 5 per second (200 msec inter-MUAP onset interval). The interpotential interval with minimum effort is best appreciated with a sweep of 100 to 200 msec/cm. *Recruitment*

Figure 18-16. *Normal motor unit recruitment with graded voluntary contraction. A. Minimal effort with an onset frequency of 5/sec. B. Recruitment of a second motor unit with increased effort—recruitment frequency of 10/sec. C–F. Increasing motor unit recruitment with a graded increase in effort leading to a complete interference pattern with maximal effort (F).*

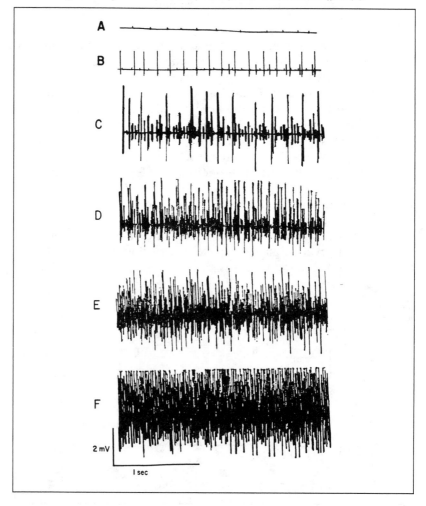

frequency is the firing rate of a motor unit action potential when a second MUAP is recruited (Fig. 18-16) and is usually 10 to 15 per second (66 to 100 msec interpotential interval). The first unit stabilizes in frequency at the moment of recruitment, and at the onset the second unit fires at a rate similar to that of the first [21]. This rate of firing can increase up to 25 to 50 per second (20 to 40 msec interpotential interval) with increased effort. The average normal onset interval is 132 msec (MUAP firing at 7.5 per second) and the average normal recruitment interval is 90 msec (original MUAP firing at 11 per second) (Table 18-10). In both myopathies and neuropathies the onset and recruitment intervals tend to be shorter [22] (Table 18-11). *Recruitment ratio* is another gauge

Table 18-10. *Onset and Recruitment Intervals in Normal Human Muscle*

Muscle	Onset intervals (mean ± SD in msec)	Recruitment intervals (mean ± SD in msec)
All facial muscles	86 ± 29	40 ± 16
Deltoid	116 ± 23	84 ± 16
Biceps	124 ± 21	86 ± 14
Triceps	132 ± 36	84 ± 17
Brachioradialis	116 ± 22	78 ± 18
Pronator teres	132 ± 38	88 ± 19
First dorsal interosseous	142 ± 39	98 ± 21
Vastus lateralis	126 ± 30	88 ± 18
Gluteus maximus	128 ± 30	88 ± 16
Tibialis anterior	124 ± 26	90 ± 13
Biceps femoris	132 ± 29	92 ± 16
Medial gastrocnemius	156 ± 29	110 ± 23
Extensor digitorum brevis	138 ± 29	98 ± 13
All muscles	132 ± 32	90 ± 19

Source: Adapted from J. H. Petajan and B. A. Philip. Frequency control of motor unit action potentials. *Electroencephalogr. Clin. Neurophysiol.* 27:66, 1969. Used by permission.

Table 18-11. *Onset and Recruitment Intervals in Neuropathy and Myopathy*

	Mean (± SD in msec)		Range (msec)
Neuropathy	OI	48 ± 17	15–110
	RI	36 ± 12	10–65
Myopathy	OI	65 ± 11	40–112
	RI	45 ± 8	20–58
Normal	OI	132 ± 32	76–236
	RI	90 ± 19	44–164

OI = onset interval; RI = recruitment interval.

Source: Adapted from J. H. Petajan. Clinical electromyographic studies of diseases of the motor unit. *Electroencephalogr. Clin. Neurophysiol.* 36:395, 1974. Used by permission.

of recruitment which is easier to measure than recruitment intervals. Recruitment ratio refers to the ratio of the motor unit firing rate to the number of active motor units present and is normally less than 5 [16]. For example, at a motor unit firing frequency of 15 Hz the ratio will be 15 if only one unit is firing, 10 if two units are firing, and 5 if three motor units are firing. A ratio greater than 5 indicates loss of motor units and is especially useful when faced with an incomplete interference pattern that is difficult to interpret.

Interference Pattern
The interference pattern is the electrical activity recorded from a muscle with a needle electrode during full effort [1]. A *full* or *complete interference pattern* implies that no individual motor unit potentials can be identified (Fig. 18-17A,B). Recruitment is said to be normal when a complete interference pattern occurs with maximal effort. The amplitude of a normal interference pattern is quite variable but is usually between 2 to 4 mV. It is measured from the envelope curves by the negative and positive peaks, excluding high solitary peaks [3]. A *reduced* or *incomplete interference pattern* is one in which some of the individual MUAPs may be identified while others cannot because of overlap (Fig. 18-17C). *Discrete pattern* implies that each of the MUAPs can be identified with rapid firing rates during maximal effort (Fig. 18-17D). Finally, the term *single unit pattern* is used to describe a single unit firing at rapid rates during maximal voluntary effort. The force of contraction associated with the different interference patterns should be specified [1].

Abnormal Patterns of Recruitment
MYOPATHIC DISORDERS. Patients with myopathic disorders have scattered single-fiber loss with relative preservation of the number of motor units. Recruitment is increased because more units need to be activated for any given effort. A full interference pattern of reduced amplitude is often seen with weak effort (see Fig. 18-17B). The contrast between the weakness of the muscle and the full recruitment at the very onset of the contraction can be very striking [3].

NEUROPATHIC DISORDERS. Patients with neuropathic disorders have a reduced number of motor units so that there is decreased recruitment, although the remaining units fire rapidly with any given effort (see Fig. 18-17C,D). The interference pattern is reduced (incomplete) or even discrete in severe cases. However, analysis of reduced interference is more difficult. Effort cannot be assumed to be full unless the rate of firing of the MUAPs is clearly rapid (20 to 50 per second).

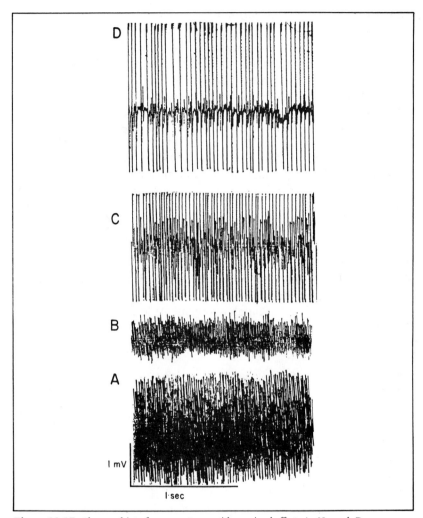

Figure 18-17. *Abnormal interference patterns with maximal effort. A. Normal. B. Myopathic—complete but of low amplitude. C. Neuropathic—reduced. D. Neuropathic—discrete.*

REDUCED ACTIVATION. Reduced activation of motor units is the inability of motor units to fire rapidly enough to recruit additional motor units when the patient voluntarily attempts to contract the muscle [18]. Reduced activation is seen with submaximal effort due to pain, fear, misunderstanding, hysteria, or malingering, or in patients with upper motor neuron weakness. The interference pattern tends to be incomplete with slow firing frequencies of MUAPs, with what seems to be maximal effort.

Analysis of Anatomic Distribution
A *myotome* is defined as a group of muscles supplied by a single spinal segment. The posterior primary ramus innervates the paraspinal muscles, and the anterior primary ramus innervates the limb muscles (Fig. 18-18). The commonly examined muscles are listed by myotome in Appendix VI. Muscles often belong to more than one myotome and most are innervated by more than one spinal segment, although the major innervation may be from one root (see Appendixes V and VI). Evaluation of several muscles in an extremity in more than one peripheral nerve and root distribution is useful for localization of an abnormality. In practice, it may at times be possible only to localize the lesion to two adjacent segments. There is considerable individual variation in the root distribution to the various muscles and some disagreement in the literature [12,15,16,19].

Paraspinal Muscles
The innervation of long paraspinal muscles is diffusely overlapped. The presence of abnormalities helps in differentiating a plexus (paraspinal sparing) from a root (paraspinal involvement) lesion, but does not help in segmental localization. The deeper, short paraspinal muscles (mul-

Figure 18-18. *Anterior and posterior rami of a spinal nerve.*

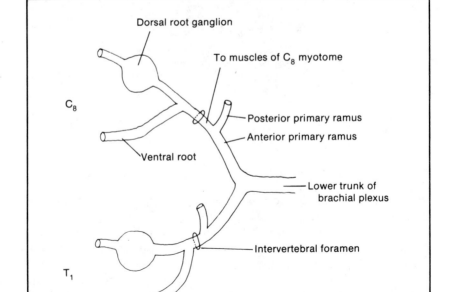

tifidus) located immediately posterior to the transverse processes are more selectively innervated by the corresponding posterior rami, but their examination is technically more demanding.

Sphincter Muscles

The anal and external urethral sphincters are innervated by the $S_{2,3,4}$ spinal nerves through the pudendal nerve. The needle insertion for the anal sphincter is about 1 cm to the side of the anal orifice. External urethral sphincter EMG is most useful when performed with a urodynamic study (Fig. 18-19). Unlike other striated muscles, the sphincters have continuous activity of motor units at rest. Relaxation of sphincter activity can be achieved by attempted micturition or defecation. The motor unit mean duration of 5.5 to 7.5 msec is shorter than in limb muscles. The *bulbocavernosus reflex* (Fig. 18-19) consists of contraction of striated pelvic floor muscles, including the sphincters, on compression or electrical stimulation of the glans penis (or clitoris). The latency of the electrically evoked response is 30 to 40 msec. The *anocutaneous reflex* tests contraction of striated sphincter muscles to mechanical stimulation of the perianal skin. These sacral segmental reflexes assess the integrity of the $S_{2,3,4}$ spinal segments and their afferent and efferent connections. They may be prolonged or absent in disorders producing lower motor neuron sacral dysfunction.

Figure 18-19. *Schematic illustration of a normal bulbocavernosus reflex (BCR) during a urodynamic study with EMG recording from the external urethral sphincter. Downward pointing arrows indicate where the BCR was elicited, and the upward pointing arrow indicates onset of voiding. Note the suppression of the BCR during voiding in normal individuals. (From R. K. Sethi et al. Modulation of the bulbocavernosus reflex during voiding: Loss of inhibition in upper motor neuron lesions. Muscle Nerve, in press. Used by permission.)*

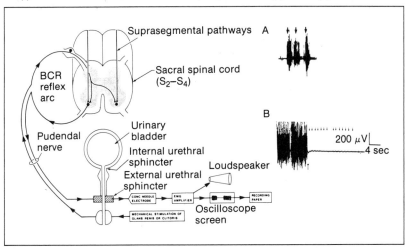

The EMG Report

The EMG report should contain the findings in each muscle tested. These findings include:

1. Insertional and spontaneous activity.
2. Characteristics of the motor unit action potentials.
3. Recruitment and interference pattern.
4. Interpretation of abnormalities—normal, myopathic, or neuropathic.

The report should next summarize the electrophysiologic findings on EMG and nerve conduction studies and give a conclusion about the type of abnormality, localization, and severity. This information should then be translated into a differential diagnosis.

References

1. AAEE glossary of terms in clinical electromyography. *Muscle Nerve* 10(8S), 1987.
2. Albers, J. W., Allen, A. A., Bastron, J. A., et al.   Limb myokymia. *Muscle Nerve* 4:494, 1981.
3. Buchthal, F.   Electromyography in the Evaluation of Muscle Disease. In M. J. Aminoff (Ed.), *Symposium on Electrodiagnosis. Neurology Clinics*. Vol. 3. Philadelphia: Saunders, 1985.
4. Buchthal, F., and Rosenfalck, P.   Action potential parameters in different human muscles. *Acta Psychiatr. Neurol. Scand.* 30:125, 1955.
5. Buchthal, F., Guld, C., and Rosenfalck, P.   Multielectrode study of the territory of a motor unit. *Acta Physiol. Scand.* 39:83, 1957.
6. Buchthal, F., and Kamieniecka, Z.   The diagnostic yield of quantified electromyography and quantified muscle biopsy in neuromuscular disorders. *Muscle Nerve* 5:265, 1982.
7. Buchthal, F., Pinelli, P., and Rosenfalck, P.   Action potential parameters in normal human muscle and their physiological determinants. *Acta Physiol. Scand.* 32:219, 1954.
8. Chokroverty, S., and Medina, J.   Electrophysiologic study of hemiplegia. *Arch. Neurol.* 35:360, 1978.
9. Daube, J. R., Kelly, J. J., and Martin, R. A.   Facial myokymia with polyradiculopathy. *Neurology* 29:662, 1979.
10. Desmedt, J. E., and Borenstein, S.   Regeneration in Duchenne muscular dystrophy: Electromyographic evidence. *Arch. Neurol.* 33:642, 1976.
11. Ekstedt, J., and Stålberg, E.   How the size of the needle lead-off surface influences the shape of the single muscle fiber action potential in electromyography. *Computer Prog. Biomed.* 3:204, 1973.
12. Goodgold, J., and Eberstein, A.   *Electrodiagnosis of Neuromuscular Diseases* (2nd Ed.). Baltimore: Williams & Wilkins, 1977.
13. Henneman, E.   Relation between size of neurons and their susceptibility to discharge. *Science* 126:1345, 1957.
14. Henneman, E., Somjen, G., and Carpenter, D. O.   Functional significance of cell size in spinal motor neurons. *J. Neurophysiol.* 28:560, 1965.
15. Johnson, E. W. (Ed.), *Practical Electromyography*. Baltimore: Williams & Wilkins, 1980.

16. Kimura, J. *Electrodiagnosis in Diseases of the Nerve and Muscle: Technique and Interpretation.* Philadelphia: Davis, 1983.
17. Licht, S. (Ed.)   *Electrodiagnosis and Electromyography* (3rd ed.). New Haven: Licht, 1971.
18. Litchy, W. J.   *Course A: Basic Nerve Conduction and Electromyography.* AAEE Ninth Annual Continuing Education Course, American Association of Electromyography and Electrodiagnosis, Boston, MA, September, 1986.
19. Liveson, J. A., and Spielholz, N. I.   *Peripheral Neurology.* Philadelphia: Davis, 1979.
20. Moersch, F. P., and Woltman, H. W.   Progressing fluctuating muscular rigidity and spasm (stiff man syndrome). *Proc. Staff Meet. Mayo Clin.* 31:421, 1956.
21. Petajan, J. H., and Philip, B. A.   Frequency control of motor unit action potentials. *Electroencephalogr. Clin. Neurophsiol.* 27:66, 1969.
22. Petajan, J. H.   Clinical electromyographic studies of the diseases of the motor unit. *Electroencephalogr. Clin. Neurophsiol.* 36:395, 1974.
23. Radu, E. W., Skorpil, V., and Kaeser, H. E.   Facial myokymia. *Eur. Neurol.* 13:499, 1975.
24. Sabra, A. F., and Hallet, M.   Action tremor with alternating activity in antagonistic muscles. *Neurology* 34:151, 1984.
25. Sacco, G., Buchthal, F., and Rosenfalck, P.   Motor unit potentials at different ages. *Arch. Neurol.* 6:44, 1962.
26. Shahani, B. T., and Young, R. R.   Physiologic and pharmacologic aids in the differential diagnosis of tremor. *J. Neurol. Neurosurg. Psychiatry.* 39:772, 1976.
27. Trojaborg, W., and Buchthal, F.   Malignant and benign fasciculations. *Acta Neurol. Scand.* 41(Suppl 13):251, 1965.
28. Trontelj, J., and Stalberg, E.   Bizarre repetitive discharges recorded with single fiber EMG. *J. Neurol. Neurosurg. Psychiatry.* 43:310, 1983.
29. Walton, J. N. (Ed.).   *Disorders of Voluntary Muscle* (3rd ed.) Edinburgh: Churchill Livingstone, 1974.
30. Warmolts, J. R., and Engel, W. K.   Open-Biopsy Electromyography. Part 1, Correlation of motor unit behavior with histochemical muscle fiber type in human muscle. *Arch Neurol.* 27:512, 1972.

Single Fiber Electromyography 19

Ekstedt and Stålberg in 1963 [2] described the technique for recording single muscle fiber action potentials using an electrode with a small (25 μm diameter) recording area. The single fiber electromyography (SFEMG) electrode is a 0.5-mm steel cannula with a central wire exposed at a side port 1 to 3 mm behind the tip (Fig. 19-1). The side port is located on the side opposite the bevelled surface (Fig. 19-1) to avoid recording from mechanically damaged fibers. A 500 to 800 Hz low-frequency filter eliminates the low frequency components from distant muscle fibers. The appropriate machine settings are given in Appendix I. The characteristics of the recorded single fiber potentials with the electrode in an optimal position are as follows [4,7].

Shape	Biphasic (initial positivity)
Duration	About 1 msec
Amplitude	Up to 25 mV (should be > 200 μV to be acceptable)
Rise time	75 to 300 μsec between positive and negative peak

Recording Technique
The extensor digitorum communis (EDC) and the frontalis are commonly used for recording. The rate of motor unit firing in these muscles can be easily controlled for the time needed to acquire a sufficient number of fiber pairs for analysis. The EDC also has the least age dependent changes [11]. The needle is inserted with the recording surface on the side port directly facing the long axis of the muscle fibers. The SFEMG recordings are usually done with mild voluntary contraction of the muscle. The needle is slowly advanced until a crisp sound is heard over the loudspeaker from a single fiber potential. In a normal extensor digitorum communis muscle, single fiber discharges are recorded in 65 to 70 percent of random insertions, and paired discharges are recorded 30 percent of the time [7,8]. The action potentials of fibers belonging to the same motor unit are always coupled to each other with a very small variability from one discharge to the next (Fig. 19-2A). The interval between a potential pair results from unequal transmission time along the nerve after it branches and along the muscle fibers from the endplates to the recording electrode (see Fig. 19-1).

Electrical stimulation can also be used for studying jitter [7,10] and is particularly useful in patients who cannot sustain a voluntary con-

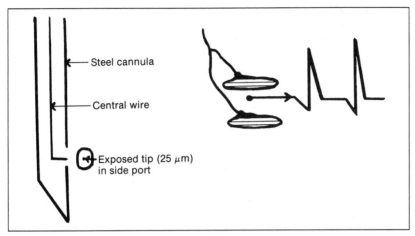

Figure 19-1. *Single fiber EMG needle* (left) *positioned between two muscle fibers* (middle) *recording the action potentials from the fiber pair* (right).

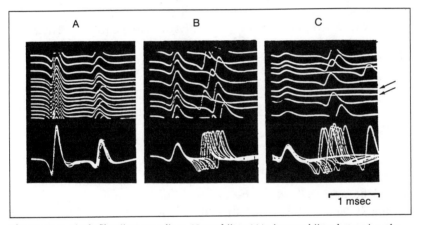

Figure 19-2. *Single fiber jitter recordings. Normal jitter* (A); *increased jitter but no impulse blocking* (B); *and increased jitter and impulse blocking* (C). *(From E. Stålberg, J. V. Trontelj, and M. S. Schwartz. Single fiber recording of the jitter phenomenon in patients with myasthenia gravis and in members of their families. Ann. N.Y. Acad. Sci. 274:192, 1976. Modified by Stålberg concerning polarity. Used by permission.)*

traction. This technique may, however, be less sensitive than voluntary activation of motor units in picking up abnormalities [10]. The main trunk of the nerve or its intramuscular branches can be stimulated. With intramuscular stimulation the cathode is a monopolar needle inserted slightly proximal to the single fiber recording electrode in the same muscle. A nearby surface disc electrode serves as the anode. Repetitive stimulation of 2 to 5 Hz is generally used, with the stimulus intensity being supramaximal for the axon to the recorded single fiber.

Single Fiber Characteristics

Two characteristics of single fibers are analyzed: the neuromuscular jitter and the fiber density.

Jitter

Jitter (Fig. 19-2) refers to the variability of the time interval between two muscle fiber action potentials belonging to the same motor unit with consecutive discharges [4,7,9]. Normal jitter is mainly due to variations in the transmission time at the two neuromuscular junctions. The jitter results from small fluctuations in the rise time of endplate potentials, which in turn reach the triggering threshold for generating a muscle fiber action potential after a variable interval [4,7,9]. *Blocking* of transmission is recognized when one member of a potential pair fails to appear intermittently (Fig. 19-2C). Blocking is usually seen when the jitter values exceed 80 to 100 μsec [7,9].

JITTER CALCULATIONS. A signal-triggered delay line and a sweep counter are used to superimpose a desired number of sweeps for analysis. The jitter is expressed as the mean consecutive difference (MCD). The MCD is the mean value of the differences between the interpotential intervals of consecutive discharges and is calculated as follows [1].

$$MCD = \frac{[D_1 - D_2] + [D_2 - D_3] + \cdots + [D_{n-1} - D_n]}{n - 1}$$

where D = individual interpotential intervals
      n = number of discharges

At least 50 discharges for each fiber pair and a minimum of 20 pairs should be analyzed when the abnormalities are minimal [1,6]. Acquiring 20 pairs requires a steady hand and a lot of patience on the part of the examiner and the patient. In practice, it is sometimes difficult to acquire 20 pairs either because of inability to maintain a steady contraction or because of difficulty with finding enough pairs [6]. Computer analysis of intervals between two potentials with an interval counter or an internal clock is the most accurate and least time consuming method [7].

For manual measurements the following procedure is followed.

1. Groups of 5 or 10 consecutive discharges are superimposed and photographed at a sweep speed of 100 to 200 μsec.
2. The range between the shortest and longest interpotential interval for the 5 (R5) or 10 (R10) superimposed single-fiber potential pairs is measured. The measurement is made close to the baseline intersection of the nontriggering potential.

3. The mean range of variations (MR5 or MR10) of interpotential intervals of the discharges is measured for at least 50 consecutive discharges (photographed in groups of 5 or 10) for each fiber pair.
4. The MCD can be calculated by multiplying the mean range for each pair (MR5 or MR10) by the appropriate factor (Table 19-1). For example, if 5 groups of 10 superimpositions are used, the mean range of variations of the interpotential interval (MR10) is multiplied by a factor of 0.37 to calculate the MCD for the pair.
5. The MCD is then determined individually for 20 different fiber pairs.
6. Finally, the average or mean MCD is determined for the 20 pairs.

The normal values of jitter for individual pairs and for all fiber pairs is given in Table 19-2. With stimulation SFEMG, the latency variability between the stimulus and the single fiber responses is calculated. Normal limits for jitter with stimulation are generally about 70 percent of those with voluntary activation.

The study is abnormal if any of the following criteria are met.

1. The mean MCD in an individual pair exceeds the normal limit for the pair in more than 10 percent of fibers (Table 19-2).
2. The mean MCD for all fiber pairs exceeds the upper normal limit (Table 19-2).
3. Blocking of transmission is seen in more than 10 percent of fiber pairs.

Table 19-1. *Conversion Factors for MCD Calculations*

Number of superimposed consecutive discharges	Conversion factor
MR5 = Mean of 5 superimposed in ten groups	0.49
MR10 = Mean of 10 superimposed in five groups	0.37

Source: Ekstedt, J., Nilsson, G., and Stålberg, E.   Calculation of electromyographic jitter. *J. Neurol. Neurosurg. Psychiatry* 37:526, 1974.

Table 19-2. *Upper Normal Limits for Jitter in Different Muscles*

Muscle	MCD for all pairs (μsec)	MCD for single fiber pair (μsec)
EDC	35	55
Biceps/deltoid	30	35
Frontalis	30	45

EDC = Extensor digitorum communis.
Source: Sanders, D. B., and Philips, L. H.   *Single Fiber Electromyography.* An AAEE Workshop, American Association of Electromyography and Electrodiagnosis, Rochester, MN, 1984.

Fiber Density

Fiber density measures the number of single fiber action potentials belonging to a motor unit that are within a 300 μm uptake radius of the recording electrode [4,7].

Recording technique for fiber density is similar to jitter measurements. The SFEMG electrode is randomly inserted into the muscle and positioned so that the triggering potential is maximized. The number of single fiber potentials discharging synchronously with the triggering potential are counted in at least 20 sites. Action potentials greater than 200 μV in amplitude and less than 300 μsec in rise time are counted to ensure that only fibers within a 300 μm radius of the triggering potential are selected [11]. A sweep speed of 0.5 msec/cm to enable a 5 msec display after the triggering potential is optimal. The fiber density is the average number of spikes recorded at 20 sites and is calculated by dividing the total number of single fiber potentials counted at all sites by the total number of sites sampled. Table 19-3 lists the normal fiber density values for different muscles and age groups.

Applications

Jitter measurement is a very sensitive but nonspecific method for evaluating neuromuscular transmission [3,5,6,9]. Table 19-4 shows the sensitivity of SFEMG in myasthenia gravis. The sensitivity increases to 94 to 99 percent [3,4,5] when testing proximal limb or cranial muscles like the frontalis. Primary disease of the nerve or muscle has to be excluded before diagnosing myasthenia gravis on the basis of jitter measurements. Increased jitter is found in neuropathies with axonal degeneration and reinnervation [12] and in some myopathies. The immature regenerating nerve terminals demonstrate pronounced neuromuscular jitter and

Table 19-3. *Normal Values: Fiber Density*

Muscle	Age (yr)			
	10–25	26–50	51–75	>75
Frontalis	1.61 ± 0.21	1.72 ± 0.21		
FDI	1.33 ± 0.13	1.45 ± 0.14		
EDC	1.47 ± 0.16	1.49 ± 0.16	1.57 ± 0.17	2.13 ± 0.41
Biceps	1.25 ± 0.09	1.33 ± 0.07		
Tibialis anterior	1.57 ± 0.22	1.56 ± 0.22	1.77 ± 0.12	
Rectus femoris	1.43 ± 0.18	1.57 ± 0.23		

EDC = extensor digitorum communis; FDI = first dorsal interosseus.
Source: From E. Stålberg and J. V. Trontelj, *Single Fiber Electromyography.* Old Woking, Surrey: Mirvalle Press, 1979.

Table 19-4. Sensitivity of Single Fiber EMG in Myasthenia Gravis

Disease severity	Percentage abnormal recording from EDC
Ocular	57
Remission	78
Generalized	87
Generalized (with EDC weakness)	100
All	84

EDC = extensor digitorum communis.
Source: Values from Sanders and Philips [4].

blocking [12]. Blocking is the electrophysiologic correlate of weakness and fatigue and indicates intermittent failure of neuromuscular transmission.

Increased fiber density is a sensitive method for detecting reinnervation and provides information analogous to type grouping in muscle biopsies. Primary muscle diseases associated with muscle fiber splitting, such as muscular dystrophies, can also cause an increase in fiber density [7].

References

1. Ekstedt, J., Nilsson, G., and Stålberg, E.   Calculation of electromyographic jitter. *J. Neurol. Neurosurg. Psychiatry* 37:526, 1974.
2. Ekstedt, J., and Stålberg, E.   A method of recording extracellular action potentials of single muscle fibers and measuring their conduction velocity in voluntary activated human muscle. *Bull. Amer. Assoc. Electromogr. Electrodiagn.* 10:16, 1963.
3. Sanders, D. B., Howard, J. F. Jr., and Johns, T. R.   Single fiber electromyography in myasthenia gravis. *Neurology* 29:68, 1979.
4. Sanders, D. B., and Philips, L. H.   *Single Fiber Electromyography.* An AAEE workshop, American Association of Electromyography and Electrodiagnosis. Rochester, MN, 1984.
5. Stålberg, E.   Clinical electrophysiology in myasthenia gravis. *J. Neurol. Neurosurg. Psychiatry* 43:622, 1980.
6. Stålberg, E., Ekstedt, J., and Broman, A.   Neuromuscular transmission in myasthenia gravis studied with single fiber electromyography. *J. Neurol. Neurosurg. Psychiatry* 37:540, 1974.
7. Stålberg, E., and Thiele, B.   Transmission block in terminal twigs: A single fiber electromyographic finding in man. *J. Neurol. Neurosurg. Psychiatry* 35:52, 1972.
8. Stålberg, E., and Trontelj, J. V.   *Single Fiber Electromyography.* Old Woking, Surrey: Mirvalle Press, 1979.
9. Stålberg, E., Trontelj, J. V., and Schwartz, M. S.   Single muscle fiber recording of the jitter phenomenon in patients with myasthenia gravis and in members of their families. *Ann. N. Y. Acad. Sci.* 274:189, 1976.

10. Schwartz, M. S., and Stålberg, E.   Single fiber electromyographic studies in myasthenia gravis with repetitive nerve stimulation. *J. Neurol. Neurosurg. Psychiatry* **38**:678, 1975.
11. Thiele, B., and Stålberg, E.   Motor unit fiber density in the extensor digitorum communis muscle: Single fiber electromyographic study in normal subjects at different ages. *J. Neurol. Neurosurg. Psychiatry* **38**:874, 1975.
12. Thiele, B., and Stålberg, E.   Single fiber EMG finding in polyneuropathy of different etiologies. *J. Neurol. Neurosurg. Psychiatry* **38**:874, 1975.

Electrodiagnosis of Specific 20
Neuromuscular Disorders

Weakness and sensory symptoms can result from central or peripheral nervous system dysfunction. *Upper motor neuron weakness* results in an inability to activate motor units, but nerve conduction studies and EMG are otherwise normal. The pathophysiologic processes in neurogenic disorders are axonal degeneration, conduction block, and conduction slowing. Conduction slowing by itself does not cause any symptoms. *Conduction block* is a failure of propagation of an action potential in spite of axonal continuity [30]. Conduction block in motor fibers causes weakness, whereas in sensory fibers it will result in decreased sensation. It can occur without any structural damage, as with the use of local anesthesia, or it can result from focal demyelination. Conduction block can be documented by demonstrating at least a 40 percent reduction in amplitude between a distal and proximal point of stimulation (Fig. 20-1). Area reduction is more accurate for documenting conduction block since temporal dispersion can also cause an amplitude reduction, but temporal dispersion is associated with an increase in duration. Axonal degeneration results in reduced size of motor and sensory responses to distal stimulation, and EMG documents evidence of denervation.

The electrophysiologic approach to the diagnosis of specific clinical disorders of the peripheral nervous system is discussed in this chapter. The abnormalities are not pathognomonic for any disease, but in conjunction with the clinical examination they provide valuable information.

Motor Neuron Diseases

Electromyography (EMG) is the single most useful test in evaluating the motor neuron diseases (Table 20-1). The diagnosis of amyotrophic lateral sclerosis (ALS) and other diffuse degenerative diseases of the anterior horn cells hinges on demonstrating widespread and progressive neurogenic changes that could not result from a focal structural spinal cord lesion. The following criteria [20,21] are useful guidelines.

1. EMG shows abnormal spontaneous activity with fibrillations, positive sharp waves, and fasciculations (see Figs. 18-5, 18-6). The motor unit

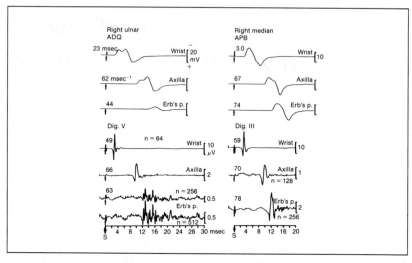

Figure 20-1. Brachial plexus lesion showing conduction block in ulnar nerve fibers. Ulnar and median nerve motor responses (above) and sensory responses (below). Latencies and conduction velocities are indicated at the traces. Note the sudden drop in motor amplitude with stimulation at Erb's point. Dispersion of the ulnar sensory response is clearly appreciated with needle electrode recording at Erb's point. (From C. Krarup and R. K. Sethi. Idiopathic brachial plexus lesion with conduction block of the ulnar nerve. Electroenceph. Clin. Neurophysiol., in press. Used by permission.)

action potentials (MUAPs) are reduced in number and increased in amplitude and duration. There is an increased incidence of polyphasic potentials (see Fig. 18-14). These abnormalities should be demonstrated in at least three extremities or in two extremities and cranial muscles such as the tongue. Two or three muscles innervated by different nerves and roots should be studied in each limb.

2. Motor conduction, including F-wave and H-reflex latencies, is either normal or shows mild slowing. Reduction of the conduction velocity is less than 40 percent of the normal mean (which can be explained by the loss of large fibers). Widespread, very low compound motor action potential (CMAP) amplitudes are poor prognostic indicators.

3. Sensory nerve conduction studies are normal.

Table 20-1. *Motor Neuron Diseases*

Diffuse degenerations (anterior horn cells)	Amyotrophic lateral sclerosis (ALS) and its variants Juvenile spinal muscular atrophy (Kugelberg-Welander's disease) Infantile spinal muscular atrophy (Werdnig-Hoffman's disease)
Focal destruction (anterior horn cells)	Infections (poliomyelitis, herpes zoster), spinal tumors, trauma, infarction, radiation, myelodysplasia, syringomyelia.

The relatively normal motor and sensory conduction velocities and late responses are important in excluding polyneuropathy or polyradiculopathy, both of which can cause widespread denervation and reinnervation. Patients with polyradiculopathy may however, have normal conduction studies. The spinal fluid protein may be raised in patients with polyradiculopathy.

Radiculopathies and Plexopathies

The relative inaccessibility of roots and plexuses makes nerve conduction studies difficult and often tends to put a greater emphasis on the needle examination [41].

Radiculopathy

Suspected root lesions from a variety of causes (Table 20-2) are one of the most common diagnoses for referral to the EMG laboratory. However, abnormalities are demonstrated in only about 50 percent of patients referred with that diagnosis [40]. Objective abnormalities on EMG may be absent if only the sensory roots are involved or if the lesion is purely demyelinating. Patients with positive EMG examinations, however, have a 70 to 95 percent correlation with myelograms [40]. Clinical and EMG abnormalities with single root lesions are generally partial because the multisegmental innervation results in an overlap of motor territories.

The following criteria are useful electrodiagnostic guidelines [40].

1. The EMG diagnosis hinges on demonstrating that any denervation activity or chronic motor unit reinnervation changes are restricted to a single root distribution. The abnormalities should be documented in at least two or more limb muscles innervated by the same root but different

Table 20-2. Radiculopathies

Cervical	Lumbosacral
Cervical spondylosis ($C_{7,6,8,5}$ in decreasing frequency)	Herniated disc (S_1, $L_{5,4}$ in decreasing frequency)
Herniated disc	Lumbosacral spondylosis
Traumatic avulsion	Multisegmental—cauda equina
Tumors—primary and metastatic	Spinal stenosis
	Tumors—primary and metastatic
	Spinal arachnoiditis
	Spinal arteriovenous malformation
	Diabetic amyotrophy

peripheral nerves and absent in muscles not innervated by that root (see Appendixes V, VI). Fibrillation potentials take 2 to 5 weeks to develop, whereas reinnervation changes take at least 6 to 8 weeks after the onset of symptoms. Neurogenic changes start in the more proximal muscles, like the paraspinal muscles, and progressively involve the more distal muscles. Reduced recruitment with increased firing frequency may be seen even before other EMG findings have developed.

2. Paraspinal muscle involvement is corroborative evidence of a proximal lesion, but their absence does not exclude a radiculopathy. Neurogenic EMG changes in paraspinal muscles are the first to appear and, in a small percentage of patients, may be restricted to those muscles. Extensive myotomal overlap in superficial paraspinals makes localization to a single root difficult. Postlaminectomy changes persist for a long time and make interpretation of any abnormalities difficult in such patients.

3. Segmental sensory stimulation of appropriate cutaneous nerves (Table 20-3) is normal in spite of any sensory loss, because with preganglionic lesions the peripheral sensory axons remain intact [5].

4. F-wave latencies are usually normal because the short involved segment is diluted by a long, normally conducting, distal segment. The H-reflex is often abnormal in S_1 root lesions.

PLEXOPATHIES. Plexopathies (Table 20-4) need to be differentiated from single or multiple radiculopathies as well as from more distal mononeuropathies.

Electrophysiologic characteristics of plexus lesions are as follows:

1. EMG evidence of denervation and/or reinnervation in more than a single root or peripheral nerve distribution.
2. Paraspinal muscle sparing.
3. Absent or reduced (<50 percent compared to the asymptomatic limb)

Table 20-3. Segmental Sensory Stimulation

Cutaneous nerve	Spinal segment
Musculocutaneous nerve	$C_{5,6}$
Median nerve (thumb)	C_6
Median nerve (middle finger)	C_7
Superficial radial nerve	$C_{6,7}$
Ulnar nerve (little finger)	C_8
Saphenous nerve	L_4
Superficial peroneal	L_5
Sural nerve	S_1

Table 20-4. *Plexus Lesions*

Brachial	Lumbosacral
Trauma	Surgical trauma, pelvic fractures
Neoplastic infiltration (lung, breast, lymphoma)	Neoplastic infiltration (lymphoma, ovarian, uterine)
Radiation	Radiation
Thoracic outlet syndrome	Retroperitoneal hemorrhage
Familial-recurrent (AD)	Psoas abscess
Idiopathic (Parsonage-Turner)	Diabetic amyotrophy
	Idiopathic

AD = autosomal dominant.

sensory nerve action potentials on appropriate segmental sensory stimulation (see Table 20-3).
4. Prolonged latencies of appropriate late responses (F-wave or H-reflex) and of motor latencies with proximal root or plexus stimulation.

In practice, it can be difficult to distinguish mild plexus lesions from root lesions. This is because (1) paraspinal denervation is not always seen with root lesions, (2) significant reduction of the sensory nerve action potential may not occur with mild partial lesions of the plexus, (3) segmental sensory evaluation of the upper brachial and lumbar plexuses is technically less reliable, and (4) lesions with pure segmental demyelination will not show reduced sensory amplitudes or evidence of denervation and can only be localized by demonstrating conduction slowing or conduction block across the involved segment (Fig. 20-1), which is technically more difficult with all proximal lesions [41].

PROGNOSIS. The overall prognosis depends on the underlying cause for the lesion. The severity in root or plexus lesions is proportional to the amount of axonal degeneration in motor and sensory fibers. The amount of axonal degeneration can be gauged by the degree of reduction in amplitudes to distal stimulation. Recovery is faster and more complete in upper brachial plexus lesions as compared to lower brachial plexus lesions. Severe preganglionic root lesions such as traumatic avulsions carry a very grave prognosis for recovery.

Entrapment Neuropathies
Mononeuropathies resulting from mechanical compression are referred to as entrapment neuropathies. The pathophysiology in entrapment neuropathies is focal demyelination [29] with secondary axonal degeneration as severity of compression increases.

Multiple entrapments can be seen in "tomaculous neuropathy," which is an autosomal dominant familial susceptibility to pressure palsies [4]. To differentiate multiple entrapments from generalized neuropathy it is important to test nerves that are not normally subject to entrapment (e.g., the superficial radial in the upper extremity).

Patients with a generalized neuropathy are also more prone to entrapments at commonly recognized entrapment sites. The electrophysiologic diagnosis of entrapment in patients with generalized neuropathies is more difficult and is established by demonstrating that the abnormality at the suspected entrapment site is out of proportion to that seen in other nerves with similar conduction characteristics.

A combination of a nerve entrapment and a radiculopathy (e.g., carpal tunnel syndrome and a C_6 or C_7 radiculopathy), each contributing partially to the symptoms, is not uncommon and is sometimes referred to as the double crush syndrome [10].

The three most common entrapment neuropathies in decreasing frequency are (1) median nerve at the wrist, or carpal tunnel syndrome (Fig. 20-2) [8,38], (2) ulnar nerve at the elbow (Fig. 20-3) [26,32], and (3) common peroneal nerve at the fibular head [35].

Electrophysiologically, entrapments are characterized by the following:

1. Focal slowing of conduction and/or conduction block is seen across the suspected site of entrapment. Sensory conduction studies across the entrapment are generally more sensitive than motor studies [8,35,38] but are technically difficult at proximal sites using surface electrodes. Slowing in motor conduction is demonstrable in only about two-thirds of patients with carpal tunnel syndrome [38], in about 50 percent of patients with an ulnar neuropathy at the elbow [32], and in only one-third of patients with a common peroneal palsy at the fibular head [35]. Conduction block is more common and more prominent in acute compression neuropathies. The chances of demonstrating focal slowing are increased by the measurement of seg-

Figure 20-2. Carpal tunnel syndrome (above) *showing a prolonged distal motor latency* (A); *slowing of sensory conduction from digit II to wrist* (B); *and slowing of mixed nerve conduction from palm to wrist* (C). *The normal tracings* (below) *are for comparison.*

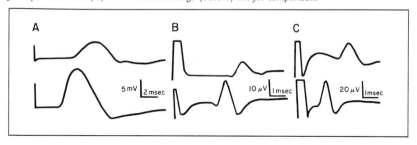

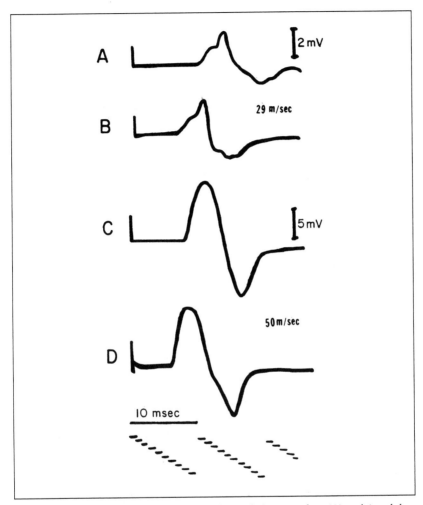

Figure 20-3. *Ulnar entrapment neuropathy with stimulation 6 cm above (A) and 4 cm below (B) the ulnar sulcus. Note the reduced motor amplitude and segmental slowing of motor conduction across the elbow. Normal ulnar nerve conduction with stimulation 6 cm above (C) and 4 cm below (D) the ulnar sulcus are shown for comparison.*

mental conduction velocity over short distances of about 10 cm across the suspected site of entrapment. Precise localization may also be accomplished with "inching" techniques where the nerve is stimulated in 1-cm intervals across the suspected entrapment [17,26]. The latency normally increases by about 0.2 msec/cm assuming a conduction velocity of 50 m/sec. A disproportionate increase in latency or evidence of a conduction block may be seen across the site of entrapment.

2. Reduced motor and sensory amplitudes to stimulation distal to the entrapment are indicators of the severity of compression since they reflect on the amount of axonal degeneration.
3. EMG evidence of denervation and/or reinnervation restricted to the muscles that are innervated by the entrapped nerve distal to the site of entrapment is seen with axonal degeneration.

Traumatic Neuropathies

Seddon [34] classified nerve injuries according to severity into three categories: neuropraxia, axonotmesis, and neurotmesis. In practice, there is overlap of these categories in individual cases. Table 20-5 lists the sequence of post-traumatic findings on electrophysiologic testing.

Neuropraxia

With neuropraxia there is immediate conduction block across the site of injury with normal conduction distally. In its mildest form there is no structural damage with rapid reversibility of symptoms, whereas with more severe trauma there is focal demyelination without interruption of axons. Recovery in the latter occurs over a few weeks during which time, slowing of the conduction velocity can be demonstrated across the lesion. EMG shows reduced recruitment of motor units when motor fibers are involved.

Axonotmesis

With axonotmesis there is interruption of axons with preservation of the nerve sheath resulting in immediate conduction failure across the site of injury. Wallerian degeneration occurs distally but conduction velocity is preserved distal to the injury site for up to 7 days [12–14]. There is a decline in the amplitude of evoked responses on distal stimulation during this first week progressing to complete failure of neuromuscular transmission. Denervation activity with fibrillations and positive sharp waves appear in the affected muscles in 2 to 5 weeks depending on the distance from the injury site. The ability to activate any motor units suggests at least partial continuity of the nerve and

Table 20-5. *Sequence of Post-Traumatic Findings*

Electrophysiologic abnormality	Timing of onset
Conduction block across injury site	Immediate
Reduced amplitudes on distal stimulation	>7 days
Denervation changes on EMG	2–5 weeks
Reinnervation on EMG (partial lesions)	>6–8 weeks

carries a better prognosis. Uncomplicated regeneration occurs at the rate of about 1 to 2 mm per day [39] often with subsequent appearance of reinnervated potentials on EMG before any clinical evidence of improvement [18].

Neurotmesis
With neurotmesis there is interruption of the axon and nerve sheath. Electrophysiologically, the findings are identical to those seen with axonotmesis, but regeneration does not occur as expected and, therefore, the nerve needs to be repaired surgically. The functional recovery, even with surgical repair, is generally poor and neuroma formation is common. The conduction velocities do not return to more than 80 percent of normal [3,7].

Electrophysiologic studies done during the first week cannot, therefore, differentiate between neuropraxia or axonal transection. Serial studies can be extremely useful for prognostication and in directing appropriate management of patients with traumatic nerve injuries.

Polyneuropathies

Electrophysiologic studies can objectively document a peripheral neuropathy, quantitate its severity, and differentiate the principal pathology—axonal degeneration or demyelination. The information acquired is useful for prognosis and in directing appropriate therapy of potentially treatable neuropathies. If a nerve biopsy is needed, nerve conduction studies help in selecting the nerve most likely to show abnormalities.

Electrophysiologic Evaluation
Electrophysiologic evaluation for peripheral neuropathies should include nerve conduction studies and electromyography.

NERVE CONDUCTION STUDIES. Nerve conduction studies of multiple sensory and motor nerves, including late responses, are performed to document abnormalities in latencies, conduction velocities and amplitudes. Sensory nerve conduction abnormalities are specific and more sensitive for polyneuropathies [22]. The abnormalities often start in the lower extremities in most axonal "dying back" neuropathies and are generally pronounced in the legs by the time the arms are involved. Abnormalities of sural sensory responses and H-reflexes occur early in the course of neuropathies and serve as useful screening tests (Fig. 20-4). If a multifocal process is suspected it can be confirmed by demonstrating asymmetric abnormalities by comparing conduction in different segments of the same nerve, in similar nerves on the two sides, and in different nerves with similar conduction characteristics.

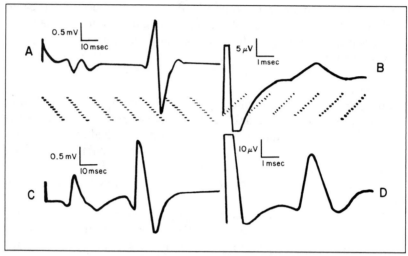

Figure 20-4. *Axonal neuropathy with a prolonged H-reflex (A) and a reduced sural sensory amplitude (B), in contrast to a normal H-reflex (C), and a normal sural sensory response (D).*

ELECTROMYOGRAPHY. EMG is performed in at least three muscles innervated by different roots and peripheral nerves in one leg and one arm to document ongoing denervation and reinnervation changes. The EMG abnormalities are of graded severity, being most prominent in the distal limb muscles and often restricted to the legs in mild neuropathies.

Pathophysiology

AXONAL NEUROPATHIES The hallmark of axonal neuropathies is reduced sensory and motor amplitudes with only mild slowing of the conduction velocities and latencies. The reduction in conduction velocity is generally less than 40 percent of the normal mean [11] (or less than 30 percent of the lower normal limit). Diabetes and alcohol abuse are the most common causes of axonal neuropathies, but the list of potential etiologies is long (Table 20-6). Most neuropathies affect motor and sensory fibers, but selective involvement of sensory fibers occurs with lesions affecting the dorsal root ganglia as well (Table 20-6).

DEMYELINATING NEUROPATHIES. The hallmark of demyelination is marked slowing of conduction velocities and latencies including those of late responses such as F-waves (Fig. 20-5). Acquired inflammatory demyelinating neuropathies (Table 20-7) have similar electrophysiologic abnormalities but are differentiated by their temporal profile into acute (eg. Guillain-Barré syndrome) or chronic. The abnormalities in Guillain-Barré syndrome are present in 50 percent of cases in the first two weeks but can be documented in 90 percent of cases in the subsequent weeks [1,24].

Table 20-6. *Axonal polyneuropathies*

Symmetric Sensorimotor	
Metabolic	Diabetes mellitus, uremia, liver disease, thyroid disease, porphyria
Toxic	Alcohol, drugs, industrial toxins
Nutritional deficiency	Thiamine, vitamin B_{12} deficiency
Paraneoplastic	Especially small cell carcinoma of lung
Dysproteinemias	Myeloma, macroglobulinemia, cryoglobulinemia, benign monoclonal gammopathy
Collagen vascular diseases	Rheumatoid arthritis, systemic lupus erythematosus, Sjögren's syndrome
Infections	Leprosy, sarcoid
Genetic	Charcot-Marie-Tooth (axonal form), familial amyloid neuropathy
Purely Sensory Neuronopathy—Dorsal Root Ganglia (DRG)	
Acute	Acute sensory neuronopathy [37] Pyridoxine toxicity
Subacute	Paraneoplastic [15]
Chronic	
Large DRG cells	Hereditary—Friedreich's ataxia (AR), abetalipoproteinemia (AR), Bassen-Kornzweig's disease), ataxia telangiectasia (AR), hereditary sensory neuropathy (AD, Denny-Brown), congenital sensory neuropathy (AR)
Small DRG cells	Fabry's disease (AR)
Multifocal Axonal	
Vasculitides	Polyarteritis nodosa, Churg-Strauss vasculitis, Wegener's granulomatosis, mixed cryoglobulinemia, Behçet disease, lupus erythematosus, rheumatoid arthritis, Sjögren's syndrome
Diabetic vasculopathy	

AD = autosomal dominant; AR = autosomal recessive.

Figure 20-5. *Guillain-Barré syndrome* (above) *with dispersion and prolonged distal latency of the median motor response* (A) *and a prolonged latency of tibial F-waves* (B). *A normal median motor response* (C) *and normal tibial F-wave latency* (D) *are shown for comparison.*

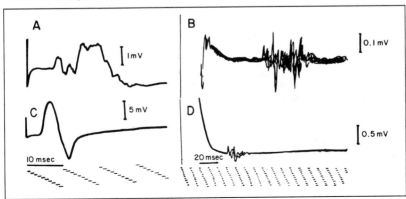

Table 20-7. *Acquired Demyelinating Neuropathies*

Acute	Chronic

1. Guillain-Barré syndrome
  a. Parainfectious
    (1) Upper respiratory infection
    (2) Gastroenteritis
    (3) Epstein-Barr virus
    (4) Cytomegalovirus
    (5) Hepatitis B
    (6) *Toxoplasma*
    (7) AIDS
  b. Post immunization
  c. Post surgery
  d. Paraneoplastic
  e. Idiopathic
2. Infections—diphtheria
3. Toxins
	1. Idiopathic
	2. Paraneoplastic
	3. Paraproteinemia
	  a. Benign monoclonal gammopathy
	  b. Myeloma—osteosclerotic
	  c. Macroglobulinemia
	4. Parainfectious—AIDS
	5. Toxins

The slowing of conduction velocity is often greater than 40 percent of the normal mean [11]. Table 20-8 lists values of nerve conduction studies which are highly suggestive of demyelination [24,25]. Immature regenerating nerve fibers can, however, have very slow conduction and dispersion of motor response, both of which are normally associated with demyelinating neuropathies.

Hereditary demyelinating neuropathies (Table 20-9) generally show uniform slowing of conduction velocity in all the nerves tested, unlike the multifocal and often asymmetric involvement in the acquired de-

Table 20-8. *Values Suggestive of Demyelinating Neuropathy*

Nerve conduction parameter	Abnormal value
Upper extremity conduction velocity	<40 m/sec
Lower extremity conduction velocity	<30 m/sec
Ulnar nerve distal motor latency	>6 msec
Median nerve distal motor latency	>7 msec
Tibial/peroneal distal motor latency	>10 msec

Table 20-9. *Hereditary Demyelinating Neuropathies*

Charcot-Marie-Tooth disease (hypertrophic form)
Dejerine-Sottas disease
Refsum's disease
Metachromatic leukodystrophy
Globoid cell leukodystrophy (Krabbe's disease)
Cockaynne's syndrome

myelinating neuropathies [23,27]. Temporal dispersion of motor responses (Fig. 20-5) and conduction block (greater than 40 percent reduction in amplitude with proximal stimulation), which are characteristic of acquired demyelinating neuropathies, are not seen in hereditary demyelinating neuropathies [23,27].

Prognosis
Denervation changes and reduced amplitudes of motor and sensory responses are proportional to the degree of axonal degeneration. Prognosis of patients with Guillain-Barré syndrome is generally favorable with 80 to 90 percent recovering without any sequelae [33]. However, patients with evidence of significant secondary axonal degeneration will take longer to recover and the recovery may not be complete. In contrast, most patients with normal motor amplitudes to distal stimulation on serial studies, will, despite severe weakness, make a rapid and substantial recovery [1]. Prognosis in patients with axonal neuropathies is related to the underlying etiology.

Neuromuscular Junction Disorders
Electrophysiologic Evaluation
Electrophysiologic testing in patients with a suspected disorder of neuromuscular transmission (Table 20-10) should include routine EMG and nerve conduction studies, repetitive nerve stimulation studies, and single fiber EMG.

NERVE CONDUCTION STUDIES AND EMG. Routine nerve conduction studies and EMG are performed to exclude a primary nerve or muscle disorder. Nerve conduction studies are normal in primary disorders of the neuromuscular junction, except for a reduced motor amplitude in myasthenic syndrome. The EMG may be normal or show small short-duration motor units. The configuration (especially amplitude) of motor units may vary with continuous firing.

Table 20-10. Neuromuscular Junction Disorders

Presynaptic	Postsynaptic
Lambert-Eaton myasthenic syndrome	Myasthenia gravis
Botulism	Neonatal myasthenia
Hypermagnesemia	Congenital myasthenia
Hypocalcemia	Penicillamine-induced myasthenia
Aminoglycosides	Aminoglycosides
Reinnervation	

REPETITIVE NERVE STIMULATION TESTING. In myasthenia gravis and other post-synaptic disorders the initial compound muscle action potential (CMAP) is of normal amplitude. The most characteristic finding is a smooth progressive decrement (of at least 10 percent) of successive action potentials until the fourth or fifth response with slow repetitive stimulation (see Fig. 17-3) [31]. Postactivation facilitation and exhaustion (see Fig. 17-4) should be demonstrated in all patients and any decrement should be reproducible. Patients with reinnervation may show changes similar to myasthenia, but these patients are easily distinguished by other electrophysiologic tests. Abnormalities on repetitive stimulation are seen in 50 to 95 percent of patients [31,36] when at least two muscles including a proximal limb or facial muscle are tested. However, if the muscle being tested is clinically weak and no decrement can be demonstrated, then the weakness is unlikely to be from myasthenia gravis.

In contrast, in patients with Lambert-Eaton myasthenic syndrome (LEMS) the baseline CMAP is consistently of low amplitude (see Fig. 17-4) and any muscle can be selected for testing. The decrement is similar to that in myasthenia gravis, but the most prominent change is the marked increment following isometric contraction or with rapid repetitive stimulation (see Figs. 17-4, 17-5) of 2 to 20 times above the baseline response. *Botulism* shows changes similar to LEMS except the postactivation facilitation is not as marked (usually less than 100 percent) and the involvement of muscles is often more selective; thus more than one site may need to be tested [9]. In infants, increments greater than 20 percent may be abnormal [19].

SINGLE FIBER EMG (SFEMG). Increased jitter and blocking (see Fig. 19-2) is seen in 94 percent of patients when the extensor digitorum and frontalis are tested [36]. SFEMG is positive in 79 percent of patients with a nondiagnostic repetitive stimulation test [16]. Abnormalities are generally more prominent in more proximal muscles and facial muscles.

Muscle Diseases

Electromyography supplements muscle enzyme tests and histology in the evaluation of patients with primary disorders of the muscles (Table 20-11). In contrast to muscle biopsy, EMG samples more sites and has a higher probability of picking up abnormalities where the disease process is patchy [6]. Muscle diseases with predominantly physiologic abnormalities, such as thyroid myopathy, show prominent abnormalities on EMG in spite of normal histology. Finally, myotonic discharges on EMG are more specific than the nonspecific histologic changes in patients with myotonic disorders.

Table 20-11. *Primary Muscle Diseases*

Hereditary	Acquired
Muscular dystrophies	Inflammatory myopathies
Duchenne's	Polymyositis/dermatomyositis
Becker	Inclusion body myositis
Fascioscapulohumeral	Infections—viral, bacterial, parasitic
Limb-girdle	Sarcoid myopathy
Ocular myopathy	Myositis ossificans progressiva
Emery-Dreifuss	
Distal myopathy (Welander)	
Myotonic disorders	Metabolic myopathies
Myotonic dystrophy	Mitochondrial myopathies
Myotonia congenita	Endocrine myopathies—thyroid, steroid
Paramyotonia congenita	Nutritional and toxic—alcohol
Metabolic	
Periodic paralysis	
Glycogen storage diseases	
Congenital myopathies	
Nemaline	
Central core	
Myotubular	
Congenital fiber type disproportion	
Congenital muscular dystrophy	

Myopathy
The diagnosis of myopathy is made on the needle examination by documenting myopathic changes in the motor units (small, short duration, polyphasic) (see Fig. 18-14). There is rapid recruitment of motor units with a complete interference pattern of reduced amplitude on weak effort (see Fig. 18-16). Fibrillations and positive sharp waves can be seen in inflammatory myopathies, muscular dystrophies, and some toxic myopathies. The diagnosis of myopathy can be documented in 87 percent of patients if quantitative methods are used [6]. Mild myopathies, especially those predominantly affecting type II fibers (e.g., steroid myopathy) are easily missed since type I fibers are the ones mainly analyzed on EMG.

MYOTONIC DISORDERS. Myotonic discharges (see Fig. 18-8) are seen in myotonia congenita, myotonic dystrophy, paramyotonia congenita, and in patients with hyperkalemic periodic paralysis. Patients with paramyotonia congenita characteristically develop a silent contracture with disappearance of the myotonic discharges on cooling the muscles by immersion in ice water for 10 minutes [28].
Nerve Conduction Studies. Nerve conduction studies are generally normal in myopathies, although a reduction in amplitudes of motor re-

sponses is possible if there has been a significant loss of muscle fibers. Patients with periodic paralysis may develop reversible inexcitability of the muscles to electrical stimulation during attacks of paralysis.

Repetitive Nerve Stimulation Testing. Repetitive stimulation in patients with myotonic disorders and periodic paralysis may show decrements which do not follow the characteristic patterns seen with neuromuscular junction disorders. With repetitive stimulation after exercise, patients with myotonia often show a decrease in amplitude (instead of facilitation), which returns to baseline after 2 to 3 minutes without any postactivation exhaustion [2].

References

1. Albers, J. W., Donofrio, P. D., and McGonagle, T. K.   Sequential electrodiagnostic abnormalities in acute inflammatory demyelinating polyradiculoneuropathy. *Muscle Nerve* 8:528, 1985.
2. Aminoff, M. J.   The declining electrical response of muscle to repetitive stimulation in myotonia. *Neurology* 27:812, 1977.
3. Ballantyne, J. P., and Campbell, M. J.   Electrophysiological study after surgical repair of sectioned human peripheral nerves. *J. Neurol. Neurosurg. Psychiatry* 36:797, 1973.
4. Behse, F., Buchthal, F., and Knappeis, G. G.   Hereditary neuropathy with liability to pressure palsy: Electrophysiologic and histopathologic aspects. *Brain* 95:777, 1972.
5. Benecke, R., and Conrad, B.   The distal sensory nerve action potential as a diagnostic tool for the differentiation of lesions in dorsal roots and peripheral nerves. *Neurology* 223:231, 1980.
6. Buchthal, F., Kamieniecka, Z.   The diagnostic yield of quantified electromyography and quantified muscle biopsy in neuromuscular disorders. *Muscle Nerve* 5:265, 1982.
7. Buchthal, F., and Kuhl, U.   Nerve conduction, tactile sensibility, and electromyogram after suture of compression of peripheral nerves: Longitudinal study in man. *J. Neurol. Neurosurg. Psychiatry* 42:436, 1979.
8. Buchthal, F., Rosenfalck, A., and Trojaborg, T.   Electrophysiologic findings in entrapment of the median nerve at the wrist and elbow. *J. Neurol. Neurosurg. Psychiatry* 37:340, 1974.
9. Cherington, M.   Electrophysiologic methods as an aid in diagnosis of botulism: A review. *Muscle Nerve* 5:528, 1982.
10. Dawson, D. M., Hallett, M., and Millender, L. H.   *Entrapment Neuropathies.* Boston: Little, Brown, 1983.
11. Gilliat, R. W.   Nerve conduction in human and experimental neuropathies. *Proc. R. Soc. Med.* 59:989, 1966.
12. Gilliat, R. W.   Recent advances in the pathophysiology of nerve conduction. In J. E. Desmedt, (Ed.), *New Developments in Electromyography and Electrophysiology.* Vol. 2. Basel: Karger, 1973.
13. Gilliat, R. W., and Hjorth, R.   Nerve conduction during wallerian degeneration in the baboon. *J. Neurol. Neurosurg. Psychiatry* 35:335, 1972.
14. Gilliat, R. W., and Taylor, J. C.   Electrical changes following section of the facial nerve. *Proc. R. Soc. Med.* 52:1000, 1959.
15. Horowich, M. S., Cho, L., and Posner, J. B.   Subacute sensory neuropathy: A remote effect of carcinoma. *Ann. Neurol.* 2:7, 1977.

16. Kelly, J. J. Jr., Daube, J. R., Lennon, V. A., et al. The laboratory diagnosis of mild myasthenia gravis. *Ann. Neurol.* 12:238, 1982.
17. Kimura, J. Localization of conduction abnormalities within the distal segment of the median nerve. *Brain* 102:619, 1979.
18. Kline, D. G., Hackett, E. R., and May P. R. Evaluation of nerve injuries by evoked potentials and electromyography. *J. Neurosurg.* 31:128, 1969.
19. Koeningsberger, M. R., Patten, B., and Lovelace, R. E. Studies of neuromuscular function in the newborn: A comparison of myoneural function in the full term and the premature infant. *Neuropaediatrie* 4:350, 1973.
20. Lambert, E. H. Electromyography in Amyotrophic Lateral Sclerosis. In F. H. Norris Jr. and L. T. Kurland (Eds.), *Motor Neuron Diseases: Research on Amyotrophic Lateral Sclerosis and Related Disorders.* New York: Grune & Stratton, 1969.
21. Lambert, E. H., and Mulder, D. W. Electromyographic studies in amyotrophic lateral sclerosis. *Proc. Mayo Clin.* 32:441, 1957.
22. Lamontagne, A., and Buchthal, F. Electrophysiologic studies in diabetic neuropathy. *J. Neurol. Neurosurg. Psychiatry* 33:442, 1970.
23. Lewis, R. A., and Sumner, A. J. The electrodiagnostic distinctions between chronic familial and acquired demyelinative neuropathies. *Neurology* 32:592, 1982.
24. McLeod, J. G. Electrophysiologic studies in Guillain-Barré syndrome. *Ann. Neurol.* 9(Suppl):20, 1981.
25. McLeod, J. G., Prineas, J. W., and Walsh, J. C. The Relationship of Conduction Velocity to Pathology in Peripheral Nerves. In J. E. Desmedt (Ed.). *New Developments in Electromyography and Electrophysiology.* Vol. 2. Karger: Basel 1973.
26. Miller, R. G. The cubital tunnel syndrome: Diagnosis and precise localization. *Ann. Neurol.* 6:56, 1979.
27. Miller, R. G., Gutmann, I., and Lewis, R. A., et al. Acquired versus demyelinative neuropathies in children. *Muscle Nerve* 8:205, 1985.
28. Nielsen, V. G., Friis, M. I., Johnsen, T. Electromyographic distinction between paramyotonia congenital and myotonia congenital: Effect of cold. *Neurology* 32:827, 1982.
29. Ochoa, J., Fowler, T. J., and Gilliat, R. W. Changes Produced by Pneumatic Tourniquet. In J. E. Desmedt (Ed.). *New Developments in Electromyography and Electrophysiology.* Vol. 2. Basel: Karger, 1973.
30. Olney, R. K., and Miller, R. G. Conduction block in compression neuropathy: Recognition and quantification. *Muscle Nerve* 7:662–667, 1984.
31. Ozdemir, C., and Young, R. R. The results to be expected from electrical testing in the diagnosis of myasthenia gravis. *Ann. N. Y. Acad. Sci.* 274:203, 1976.
32. Payan, J. Electrophysiologic localization of ulnar nerve lesions. *J. Neurol. Neurosurg. Psychiatry.* 32:208, 1969.
33. Ropper, A. H., and Shahani, B. T. Diagnosis and management of acute areflexic paralysis with emphasis on Guillain-Barré syndrome. In A. K. Asbury and R. W. Gilliat (Eds.). *Peripheral Nerve Disorders.* Boston: Butterworths, 1984.
34. Seddon, H. *Surgical Disorders of Peripheral Nerves.* Edinburgh: Churchill Livingstone, 1975.
35. Singh, N., Behse, F., and Buchthal, F. Electrophysiologic study of peroneal palsy. *J. Neurol. Neurosurg. Psychiatry.* 37:1202, 1974.
36. Stålberg, E. Clinical electrophysiology of myasthenia gravis. *J. Neurol. Neurosurg. Psychiatry.* 43:622, 1980.

37. Sterman, A. B., Schaumburg, H. H., and Asbury, A. K.   The acute sensory neuronopathy: A distinct clinical entity. *Ann. Neurol.* 7:354, 1980.
38. Steven, J. C.   AAEE minimonograph #26: The electrodiagnosis of carpal tunnel syndrome. *Muscle Nerve* 10:99, 1987.
39. Sunderland, S.   *Nerves and Nerve Injuries.* Edinburgh: Churchill Livingstone, 1978.
40. Wilbourne, A. J.   The Value and Limitations of Electromyographic Examination in the Diagnosis of Lumbosacral Radiculopathy. In R. Hardy (Ed.). *Lumbar Disc Disease.* New York: Ravens Press, 1982.
41. Wilbourne, A. J.   Electrodiagnosis of plexopathies. In M. J. Aminoff (Ed.). *Symposium on Electrodiagnosis. Neurology Clin.* 3:495, 1985.

Appendixes

Machine Settings for EMG and *I* Nerve Conduction Studies

Setting	Sweep velocity (msec/division)	Sensitivity (μv/division)	Filters high/low (kHz/Hz)	Stimulator duration/rate (msec/Hz)
Motor NCS	2	5000	10 kHz/2 Hz	0.2 msec/1 Hz
Sensory NCS	1	10	2 kHz/20 Hz	0.1 msec/2.0 Hz
H-Reflex	10	500	10 kHz/20 Hz	1 msec/0.5 Hz
F-Wave	10	500	10 kHz/20 Hz	0.2 msec/1.0 Hz
EMG				
Minimal contraction	10	100	10 kHz/10 Hz	Off
Maximal contraction	10	1000	10 kHz/10 Hz	Off
SFEMG	0.2–0.5	200	32 kHz/500 Hz	Off
Tremor study	200	200	32 kHz/500 Hz	Off
Blink reflex	5–10	200	10 kHz/20 Hz	0.05 msec/0.2 Hz
Sympathetic skin response	500	200	2 kHz/0.5 Hz	0.2 msec/0.2 Hz

Normal Values: *II*
Adults

Nerve	Lower normal limits		Upper limit of distal latency (msec)
	Maximum CV (m/sec)	Amplitude (peak to peak)	
Ulnar (motor)			
Wrist to ADQ (7.0 cm)	—	5 mV	3.0
Below elbow to wrist	51	—	—
Above elbow to wrist	51	—	—
Across extended elbow	44	—	—
Axilla to above elbow	56	—	—
Erb's point to axilla	55	—	—
Erb's point to above elbow	52	—	—
F-wave (wrist–ADQ)	—	—	32
Ulnar (sensory)			
Orthodromic (14 cm)	50	5 μV	3.2 (peak)
Median (motor)			
Wrist to APB (6.5 cm)	—	5 mV	3.8
Elbow to wrist	50	—	—
Axilla to elbow	57	—	—
Erb's point to axilla	57	—	—
Erb's point to elbow	53	—	—
F-wave (wrist–APB)	—	—	31
Median (sensory)			
Orthodromic (14 cm)	51	10 μV	3.5 (peak)
Radial (motor)			
Forearm to EIP (6.2 cm)	—	—	2.9
Elbow to EDC (11 cm)	—	7 mV	3.6
Elbow to forearm	52	—	—
Axilla to elbow	58	—	—
Erb's point to elbow	56	—	—
Radial (sensory)			
Antidromic (14 cm)	50	15 μV	3.3 (peak)
Musculocutaneous (sensory)			
Antidromic (12 cm)	57	12 μV	2.6 (peak)
Sciatic (motor)			
Gluteal fold to popliteal fossa	45	—	—
Peroneal (motor)			
Ankle to EDB (9 cm)	—	4 mV	5.0
Above fibula head to ankle	44	—	—
Below fibula head to ankle	43	—	—
Across fibula Head	41	—	—
F-wave (ankle–EDB)	—	—	57

| Nerve | Lower normal limits | | Upper limit of distal latency (msec) |
	Maximum CV (m/sec)	Amplitude (peak to peak)	
Superficial peroneal (sensory)			
Antidromic (12 cm)	40	5 μV	3.5 (peak)
Tibial (motor)			
Ankle to AH (10 cm)	—	5 mV	5.1
Ankle to ADQ (10 cm by caliper)	—	—	5.8
Popliteal fossa to ankle	43	—	—
F-wave (ankle–AH)	—	—	57
Sural (sensory)			
Antidromic (14 cm)	40	5 μV	4.4 (peak)
Medial Plantar (mixed)			
Orthodromic (14 cm)	—	10 μV	3.7 (peak)
Femoral (motor)			
Inguinal region to VM (14 cm)	—	—	4.2
Inguinal region to VM (28 cm)	—	—	6.7
CV between recording sites	50	—	—
Saphenous (sensory)			
Antidromic lower leg (14 cm)	—	2.2 μV	4.4
H-reflex			
Popliteal fossa to soleus	—	—	35
Facial (motor)			
Mastoid-nasalis (<13 cm)	—	—	4.2

ADQ = abductor digiti quinti; APB = abductor pollicis brevis; EIP = extensor indicis proprius; EDC = extensor digitorum communis; EDB = extensor digitorum brevis; AH = abductor hallucis; VM = vastus medialis.

III Normal Values: Children

Nerve	Lower normal limits		Amplitude (peak to peak)	Upper limit		Reference
	Maximum CV (m/sec)			M-wave latency (msec)	F-Wave latency (msec)	
	Newborn	1–2 yr				
Ulnar (motor)						
Wrist to ADQ						[4]
Newborn (1.9–3.4 cm)	—	—	1.6 mV	2.9	17	
1–2 yr (2.4–4.8 cm)	—	—	2.6 mV	2.2	17	
Elbow to wrist	22.4	39.2	—	—	—	
Ulnar (mixed)						[2]
Wrist to elbow	25.9	44.6	—	—	—	
Median (motor)						[4]
Wrist to APB						[4]
Newborn (1.9–3.0 cm)	—	—	2.6 mV	2.9	18.8	[4]
1–2 yr (2.2–4.3 cm)	—	—	3.7 mV	2.8	18	[4]
Elbow to wrist	20	41.3	—	—	—	
Median (sensory)						[4]
Newborn (3.8–5.4 cm)	25.1	—	8 µV	3.0 (peak)	—	
1–2 yr (5.7–9.1 cm)	—	46.5	7 µV	3.0 (peak)	—	
Median (mixed)						[2]
Wrist to elbow	23	47.5	—	—	—	

						Ref
Peroneal (motor)						[4]
Ankle to EDB						
Newborn (1.9–3.8 cm)	—	—	1.8 mV	3.1	25	
1–2 yr (2.2–5.8 cm)	—	—	1.7 mV	3.5	26	
Fibular head to ankle	21	39.2	—	—	—	
Tibial (motor)						[4]
Ankle to AH						
Newborn (1.9–3.8 cm)	—	—	—	4.2	—	
1–2 yr (2.2–5.8 cm)	—	—	—	3.0	26	
Popliteal fossa to ankle	20	35	—	—	—	
Sural (sensory)						[4]
Newborn (5.5 cm)	—	—	8 μV	3.3 (peak)		
1–2 yr (4.5–8.6 cm)	—	—	8 μV	3.0 (peak)		
Medial plantar (mixed)						[4]
Newborn (4.4–5.8 cm)	—	—	10 μV	3.3 (peak)		
1–2 yr (6.1–9.3 cm)	—	—	15 μV	2.5 (peak)		
Facial (motor)						
To orbicularis oculi						
Newborn	—	—	—	4.2		[3]
1–2 yr	—	—	—	3.7		[1]
Blink reflex						
Newborn (R_1)	—	—	—	14		[3]
Ipsilateral R_2	—	—	—	41		[3]
1–2 yr (R_1)	—	—	—	13.5		[1]

ADQ = abductor digiti quinti; APB = abductor pollicis brevis; EDB = extensor digitorum brevis; AH = abductor hallucis.

References

1. Clay, S. A., and Ramseyer, J. C.   The orbicularis oculi reflex in infancy and childhood. *Neurology* 26:521, 1976.
2. Cruz Martinez, A., Conde, P., del Campo, F., et al.   Sensory and mixed conduction velocity in infancy and childhood: Normal parameters in median, ulnar and sural nerves. *Electromyogr. Clin. Neurophysiol.* 18:487, 1978.
3. Kimura, J., Bodensteiner, J., and Yamada, T.   Electrically elicited blink reflex in normal neonates. *Arch. Neurol.* 34:246, 1977.
4. Miller, R. G., and Kuntz, N. L.   Nerve conduction studies in infants and children. *J. Child. Neurol.* 1:19, 1986.

Durations of selected CMAPs IV (msec)

Median	15.7 ± 2.4 SD
Ulnar	14.0 ± 2.14 SD
Deep peroneal	14.9 ± 3.3 SD

Source: Adapted from B. G. B. Christie and E. N. Coomes, Normal variations of nerve conduction in three peripheral nerves. *Ann. Phys. Med.* 5:303, 1959–1960. Used by permission.

The Innervation of Commonly *V* Studied Muscles by Named Nerves and Spinal Segments

Muscle	Nerve	Segment
Gluteus maximus	Inferior gluteal	$L_5, S_{1,2}$
Gluteus medius/minimus	Superior gluteal	$L_{4,5}, S_1$
Tensor fascia lata	Superior gluteal	$L_{4,5}, S_1$
Adductor of thigh	Obturator	$L_{2,3,4}$
Quadriceps femoris	Femoral	$L_{2,3,4}$
Iliopsoas	Femoral	$L_{2,3,4}$
Biceps femoris	Sciatic trunk	$L_5, S_{1,2}$
Semimembranosus	Sciatic trunk	$L_5, S_{1,2}$
Semitendinosus	Sciatic trunk	$L_5, S_{1,2}$
Tibialis anterior	Deep peroneal	$L_{4,5}$
Gastrocnemius	Posterior tibial	$S_{1,2}$
Soleus	Posterior tibial	$S_{1,2}$
Peroneus longus/brevis	Superficial peroneal	L_5, S_1
Tibialis posterior	Posterior tibial	L_5, S_1
Extensor digitorum brevis	Deep peroneal	L_5, S_1
Intrinsic foot muscles	Posterior tibial	$S_{1,2}$
Trapezius	Spinal accessory	$C_{3,4}$
Rhomboideus	Dorsal scapular	C_5
Serratus anterior	Long thoracic	$C_{5,6,7}$
Supraspinatus	Suprascapular	$C_{5,6}$
Infraspinatus	Suprascapular	$C_{5,6}$
Deltoid	Axillary	$C_{5,6}$
Biceps	Musculocutaneous	$C_{5,6}$
Brachioradialis	Radial	$C_{5,6}$
Supinator	Radial	$C_{6,7}$
Triceps	Radial	$C_{7,8}$
Extensor digitorum communis	Radial	$C_{7,8}$
Extensor indicis proprius	Radial	$C_{7,8}$
Extensor carpi radialis longus	Radial	$C_{6,7}$
Flexor carpi ulnaris	Ulnar	$C_{7,8}$
Flexor carpi radialis	Median	$C_{6,7}$
Pronator teres	Median	$C_{6,7}$
Flexor pollicis longus	Median	$C_{7,8}$
Opponens pollicis	Median	C_8, T_1
Abductor pollicis brevis	Median	C_8, T_1
Abductor digiti quinti	Ulnar	C_8, T_1
First dorsal interosseous	Ulnar	C_8, T_1

Myotomes of the Upper and **VI**
Lower Extremities

L_2 *Myotome*
Adductors of thigh
Quadriceps femoris
Iliopsoas

L_3 *Myotome*
Adductors of thigh
Quadriceps femoris
Iliopsoas

L_4 *Myotome*
Gluteus medius/minimus
Adductors of thigh
Quadriceps femoris
Tibialis anterior
Tensor fascia lata
Iliopsoas

L_5 *Myotome*
Gluteus maximus
Gluteus medius/minimus
Tensor fascia lata
Semimembranosus
Semitendinosus
Tibialis anterior
Gastrocnemius
Peroneus longus/brevis
Tibialis posterior
Extensor digitorum brevis

S_2 *Myotome*
Gluteus maximus
Gluteus medius/minimus
Biceps femoris
Gastrocnemius
Soleus
Peroneus longus/brevis
Tibialis posterior
Extensor digitorum brevis
Intrinsic foot muscles

S_2 *Myotome*
Gluteus maximus
Medial/lateral hamstrings
Gastrocnemius
Intrinsic foot muscles
Anal/external urethral sphincters

S_3 *Myotome*
Anal/external urethral sphincters

$C_{3,4}$ *Myotome*
Trapezius
Diaphragm

C_5 *Myotome*
Rhomboideus
Supraspinatus
Infraspinatus
Deltoid
Biceps
Brachioradialis
Teres major/minor

C_6 *Myotome*
Serratus anterior
Supraspinatus
Infraspinatus
Deltoid
Biceps
Flexor carpi radialis
Supinator
Pronator teres
Extensor carpi radialis longus
Brachioradialis

C_7 *Myotome*
Serratus anterior
Triceps
Extensor digitorum communis
Supinator
Flexor carpi ulnaris
Flexor carpi radialis
Pronator teres

C_8 *Myotome*
Flexor digotorum profundus
Flexor pollicis longus
Extensor digitorum communis
Extensor indicis proprius
Flexor carpi ulnaris
Triceps
Opponens pollicis
Abductor pollicis brevis
Abductor digiti quinti
First dorsal interrosseous

T_1 *Myotome*
Abductor pollicis brevis
First dorsal interosseous
Abductor digiti quinti
Opponens pollicis

Motor Points of Commonly VII
Studied Muscles

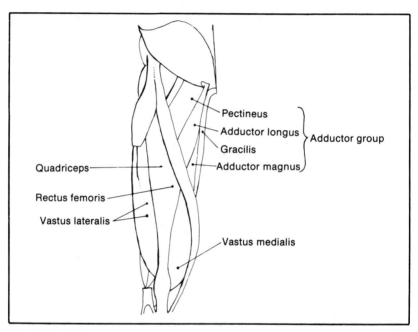

The anterior thigh.

Illustrations redrawn from S. Licht (Ed.). *Electrodiagnosis and Electromyography* (3rd ed.). New Haven: Licht, 1971.

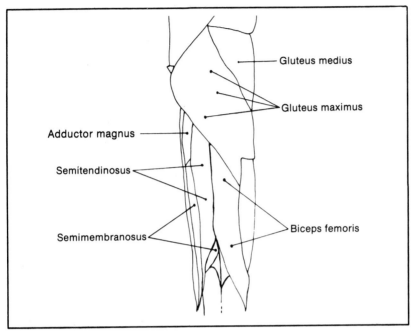

The posterior thigh.

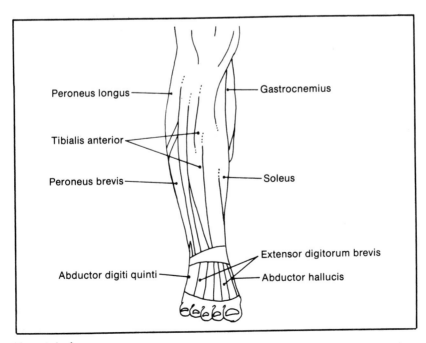

The anterior leg.

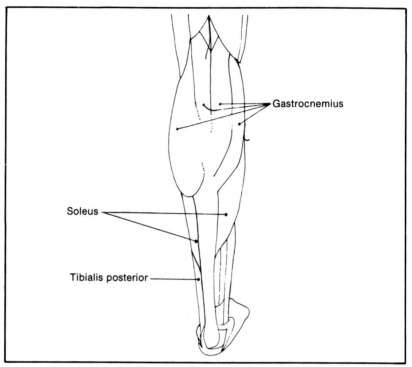

The posterior leg.

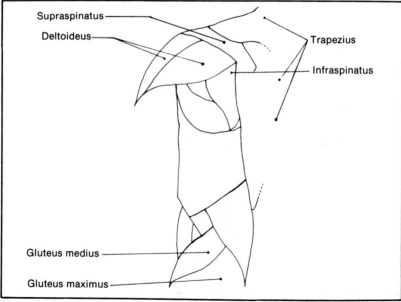

The posterior trunk.

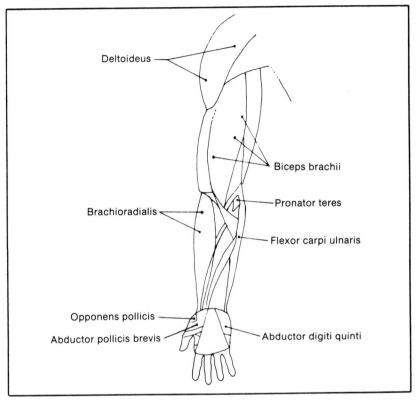

The anterior upper extremity.

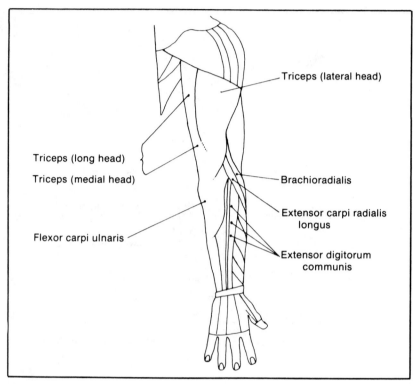

The posterior upper extremity.

Index

Index

Acetylcholine (Ach), 114–115
Acoustic neuroma, 98
Active recording electrode, 1, 4
Adductor's canal (Hunter's canal), 89
Alcohol abuse, 168
Amplifiers, differential, 5–6
Amplitude, 5–6. *See also under normal values for specific studies and procedures*
Amyotrophic lateral sclerosis (ALS), 160
Anocutaneous reflex, 149
Anode, 1, 4
Anterior interosseous nerve, 41
Anterior interosseous nerve syndrome, 42
Axonal neuropathies, 168
Axonotmesis, 166–167

Blink reflex
  anatomy of, 96
  applications for, 96–99
  normal values of, 99
  procedure for, 99
Blocking, neuromuscular, 154, 155, 156–157, 172
Botulism, 116, 143, 172
Brachial plexus motor studies
  anatomy of, 22
  applications for, 22
  conduction velocities of, 29
  latencies of from Erb's Point, 28
  procedure for, 23–29
  and axillary stimulation, 29
  and stimulation of brachial plexus, 26–28
  and stimulation of cervical root, 27, 28–29
  normal values of, 28
Bulbocavernosus reflex, 149

Canal of Guyon, 31
Carpal tunnel syndrome, 41, 164
Cathode, 1, 4
CMAP. *See* Compound muscle action potential
CNAP. *See* Compound nerve action potential
Common peroneal nerve, 67

Complex repetitive discharges (CRDs), 131
Compound muscle action potential (CMAP), 9–10, 114–115, 119, 121, 160, 172
  durations of selected, 185
Compound nerve action potential (CNAP), 17
Conduction block, motor fiber, 159, 163, 164
Conduction velocity (CV), 13–14, 17, 165, 167, 170. *See also under normal values for specific studies and procedures*
Contracture, 134
Cramps, 134
CV. *See* Conduction velocity

Decrement (repetitive stimulation), 119, 172, 174
Deep peroneal nerve, 67
Demyelinating neuropathy, acquired and hereditary, 85, 92, 98–99, 168–171. *See also* Guillain-Barré syndrome
Diabetes, 168. *See also* Ischemic mononeuropathy, diabetes
Digital signal averager, 6–7
Display screen (Cathode Ray Oscilloscope), 6
Distal motor latency, 11
Dorsal cutaneous branches (superficial peroneal nerve), 72
Dorsal sensory branch (ulnar nerve), 31, 38–39
Durations of selected CMAPs, 185

Electrodes, 1–4. *See also* Recording electrodes
Electromyography. *See* EMG, examination by
Electromyography (EMG) machine, 2, 6–7
EMG, examination by
  and analysis of anatomic distribution, 148–149
  anatomy and physiology of, 123
  and entrapment neuropathies, 163–165

EMG—*Continued*
  exertional activity in, 136–148
  insertional activity in, 126
  machine settings for, 179
  and motor neuron diseases, 159–161
  and muscle diseases, 172–174
  and neuromuscular junction disorders,
    171–172
  and plexopathy, 162–163
  and polyneuropathy, 168–171
  and radiculopathy, 161–162
  recording electrodes in, 123–125
    concentric (coaxial), 125
    monopolar, 125
  report of, 150
  single fiber. *See* Single fiber
    electromyography (SFEMG)
  spontaneous activity in, 126–136
    abnormal, 127–136
    normal, 126–127
  and traumatic neuropathies, 166–167
Endplate noise, 126
Endplate potentials (EPP), 114
Endplate spikes, 126–127
Erb's point, 23, 26, 27
Essential tremor, 135
Extensor digitorum communis (EDC),
  152

F-persistence, 101
F-wave
  anatomy and physiology of, 101
  applications for, 102
  and H-reflex, 107–109
  and motor neuron diseases, 160
  normal values of, 105
  and plexopathy, 163
  procedure for, 102–105
  and radiculopathy, 162
Facial nerve direct stimulation
  anatomy of, 92
  applications for, 92–93
  normal values of, 96
  procedure for, 93–95
Facial nerve palsy, 92
Fasciculation, 129–131, 160
Femoral nerve motor studies
  anatomy of, 83–84
  applications of, 84–85
  procedure for
    motor, 85–86
      normal values for, 87
    nerve conduction velocity between
      two points, 88
      normal values for, 87
Fiber density, 156
Fibrillation, 127–129, 160, 162, 166, 173
Filters, 6
Flexor carpi ulnaris (cubital tunnel), 31

Geniculate herpes zoster (Ramsey Hunt
  syndrome), 92
Ground electrode, 1
Guillain-Barré syndrome, 92, 168, 171.
  See also Demyelinating neuropathy,
  acquired and hereditary

H-reflex
  anatomy and physiology of, 107–109
  applications for, 109
  and motor neuron diseases, 160
  normal values of, 111–113
  and plexopathy, 163
  and polyneuropathy, 167
  procedure for, 109–110
  and radiculopathy, 162

Innervation of commonly studied muscles
  by named nerves and spinal
  segments, 186
Innervation ratio, 123
Interference pattern, 146
Ischemic mononeuropathy, diabetic, 59,
  84, 92
Ischemic femoral mononeuropathy, 84

Jitter, 153–155, 172
  calculation of, 154–155

Lambert-Eaton myasthenic syndrome
  (LEMS), 116, 119, 143, 172
Lateral antebrachial cutaneous nerve, 56
Lateral dorsal cutaneous branch (sural
  nerve), 80
Lateral epicondylitis ("resistant tennis
  elbow"), 49
Leptomeningeal carcinomatosis, 92
Ligament of Struther's syndrome, 41
LOAF muscles of the hand, 41
Loudspeaker, 6
Lumbosacral roots motor studies
  anatomy and application of. *See* Sciatic
    nerve motor studies
  procedure for, 64–65
    normal values for, 64
Lyme disease, 92

M-wave, 10, 101
Machine settings for EMG and nerve
  conduction studies, 179
Martin-Gruber anastomosis, 45
Mean consecutive difference (MCD),
  154–155
Median nerve motor and sensory studies
  anatomy of, 41–42
  applications for, 41
  and the Martin-Gruber anastomosis, 45
  procedure for
    antidromic sensory, 46–47
      normal values for, 47

motor, 42–45
normal values for, 44
median mixed nerve conduction
studies, 47
normal values for, 47
orthodromic sensory, 45–46
normal values for, 46
Metal disc and ring electrodes, 1, 2–3
Miniature endplate potentials (MEPP),
114
Motor neuron diseases and EMG, 160–
161
Motor points of commonly studied
muscles, 189–193
Motor unit, 123
Motor unit action potential (MUAP), the
abnormalities in, 142–144
amplitude of, 139
duration of, 139
and firing pattern, 144–146
and interference pattern, 146
and motor neuron diseases, 159–161
phase of, 139
physiologic variables in, 141–142
rise time of, 139
MUAP. *See* Motor unit action potential
(MUAP)
Muscle fiber action potential, 114
Muscle fibers, types I and II, 123
Muscular diseases, 172–174
Muscular dystrophy, 157, 173
Musculocutaneous nerve sensory studies
anatomy of, 56
applications for, 56
normal values of, 58
procedure for, antidromic, 56, 58
Myasthenia gravis, 116, 119, 156, 172
Myokymia, 132–134
Myopathic disorders, 142–143, 146, 172,
173
and abnormality of MUAP, 142–143
and abnormality of recruitment, 146
and nerve conduction studies, 173–174
and repetitive nerve stimulation testing,
174
Myotomes, 148
of the upper and lower extremities,
187–188
Myotonic discharges, 131–132, 173, 174

Needle electrodes, 4
Nerve conduction studies. *See also under
specific studies*
apparatus for, 1–8
experimental errors in, 20–21
general considerations in, 8–9
machine settings for, 179
mixed, 15, 17

motor, 9–14
and amplitude measurement, 10, 14
and compound muscle action
potential (CMAP), 9–10
and conduction velocity, 13–14
and dispersion of compound motor
action potential, 14
and duration and shape of response,
10, 14
and motor latency, 11–14
and neuromuscular junction disorders,
171
normal values for, 19–20
and polyneuropathies, 167
sensory, 10–14
and amplitude measurement, 16, 17
antidromic, 4, 15, 16
and compound nerve action potential
(CNAP), 16, 17
and conduction velocity, 17
orthodromic, 16
and sensory latency, 16, 17
sympathetic skin response (SSR),
18–19
and temperature, 20
and variation in conduction velocity, 20
Nerve conduction velocity (NCV). *See*
Conduction velocity (CV)
Neuromuscular junction disorders and
EMG
and nerve conduction studies, 171
and repetitive nerve stimulation testing,
172
and SFEMG, 172
Neuromyotonic discharges, 134
Neuropathies
and abnormality of MUAP, 143
and abnormality of recruitment, 146
axonal, 168
demyelinating, 168–171
entrapment, 163–166
polyneuropathy, 167–171
traumatic, 166–167
Neuropraxia, 166
Neurotmesis, 167
Normal values, nerve
adult, 180–181
child, 182–183

Onset frequency, firing pattern, 144

Paraspinal muscles, 148–149, 162
Parkisonian tremor, 135
Periodic paralysis, 173–174
Peroneal nerve motor studies
anatomy of, 67
applications of, 67
procedure for, 67–71
normal values of, 70

Physiologic tremor, 135
Plantar nerves, 78, 79
Plexopathies, 162–163
Plexus motor studies. *See* Sciatic nerve motor studies
Polyneuropathies
  and EMG, 168
  and nerve conduction studies, 167
  pathophysiology of, 168–171
Positive sharp waves, 128–129, 159, 166
Postactivation exhaustion (repetitive stimulation), 121
Postactivation facilitation (repetitive stimulation), 115, 119–120
Posterior interosseous nerve, 49
Posterior interosseous syndrome, 49
Pronator syndrome, 41

Radial nerve motor and sensory studies
  anatomy of, 49
  applications of, 49–50
  procedure for
    antidromic sensory, 53–54
      normal values for, 54
    motor, 50–52
      normal values for, 52
Radiculopathy, 161–162
Recording apparatus, 7
Recording electrodes, 123–125
Recruitment, 144–146
  abnormal patterns of, 146–147
  frequency, 144–145
  ratio, 145–146
Reduced activation, motor unit, 147
Reference electrodes, 1
Repetitive stimulation
  anatomy and physiology of, 114–115
  applications for, 116
  and myopathy, 174
  and neuromuscular junction disorders, 172
  procedure for, 116–121
    and decrement, 119
    and postactivation exhaustion, 121
    and postactivation facilitation, 119–120
    and site selection, 116
    and technical considerations to prevent artifactual changes, 116–117
    test, 117–118
Retroperitoneal hematoma, 84
Rubral (cerebral outflow) tremor, 135–136

Saphenous nerve sensory studies
  anatomy of, 89

applications for, 89
  normal values of, 91
  procedure for, antidromic sensory, 89
Sarcoidosis, 92
Satellite potentials, 139, 149
Sciatic nerve motor studies
  anatomy of, 59
  applications for, 59
  procedure for, 60–63
  normal values for, 63
Serrated potentials, 139
SFEMG. *See* Single fiber electromyography (SFEMG)
Shortest latency (F-wave), 101
Single fiber electromyography (SFEMG)
  characteristics of, 152
  electrode for, 152
  and neuromuscular junction disorders, 172
  recording technique for, 152–153
  and single fiber characteristics, 154–156
    density, 156
    jitter, 154–155
Skin temperature controlling unit, 8
Sphincter muscles, 149
Spinal nerves, 59
Spiral groove, 49
Stiff-man syndrome, 134
Stimulator, 2, 4–5
Stimulus artifact, 5
Superficial peroneal division, 67
Superficial peroneal nerve sensory studies
  anatomy of, 72–73
  applications of, 73
  normal values of, 73
  procedure for, 73
Superficial radial nerve, 49
Supinator muscle (arcade of Frohse), 49
Sural nerve sensory studies
  anatomy of, 80
  applications of, 81–82
  normal values for, 82
  and polyneuropathies, 167
  procedure for, antidromic sensory, 82
Sympathetic skin response (SSR), 18–19

Tarsal tunnel syndrome, 73
Tibial nerve motor and sensory studies
  anatomy of, 73
  applications of, 73
  procedure for
    motor, 75, 77
      normal values for, 78
    plantar nerves: mixed nerves (orthodromic), 77, 79
      normal values for, 79
Tremor studies (EMG), 135–136
Turns, EMG wave, 139

Ulnar nerve motor and sensory studies
  anatomy of, 31, 32
  applications for, 31
  procedure for
    antidromic sensory, 37
      normal values of, 37
    dorsal cutaneous branch, 38–39
      normal values of, 39

    mixed nerve conduction studies, 38
      normal values of, 38
    motor, 31–35
      normal values of, 35
    orthodromic sensory, 36
      normal values of, 36
Ulnar sulcus, 31
Upper motor neuron weakness, 159